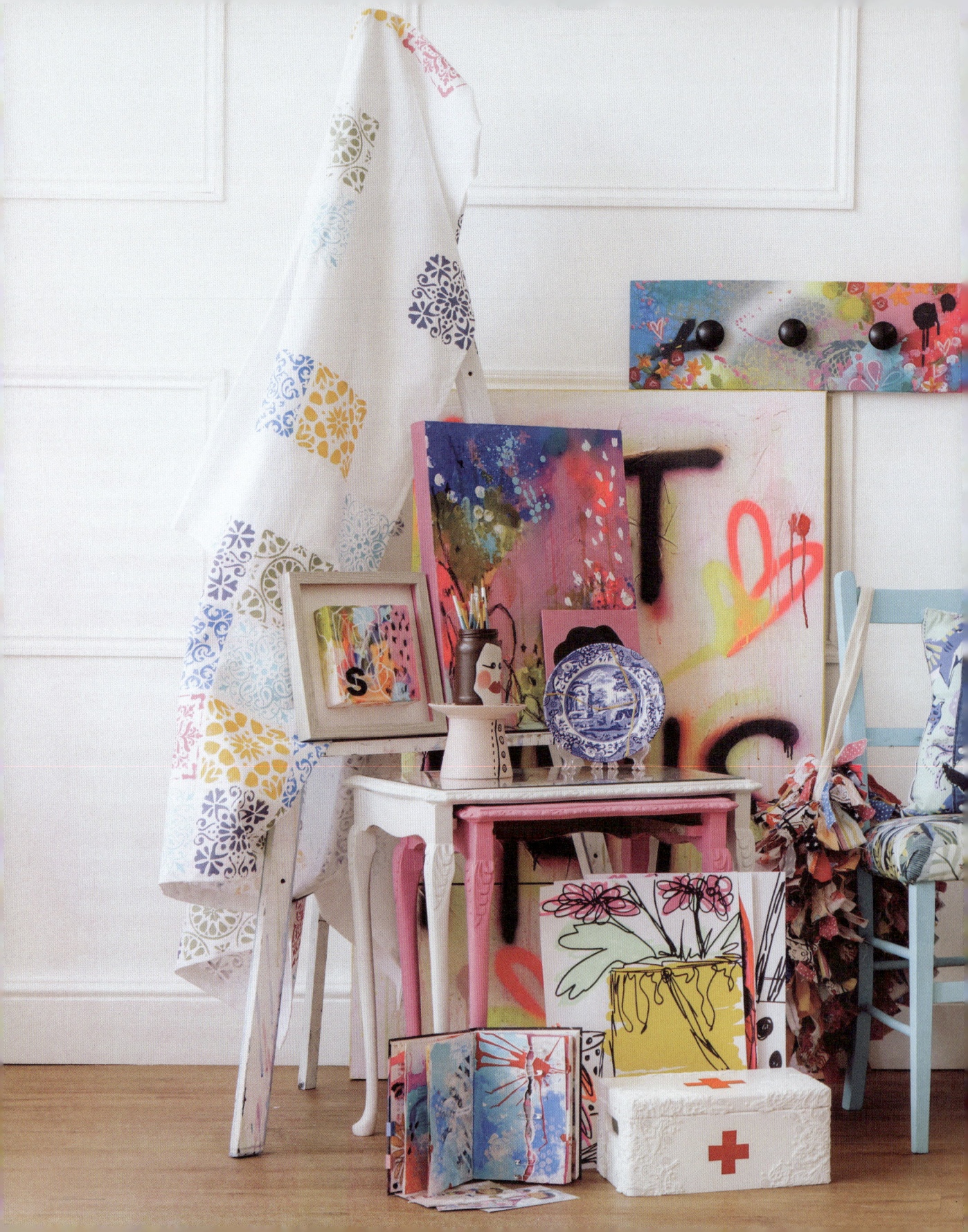

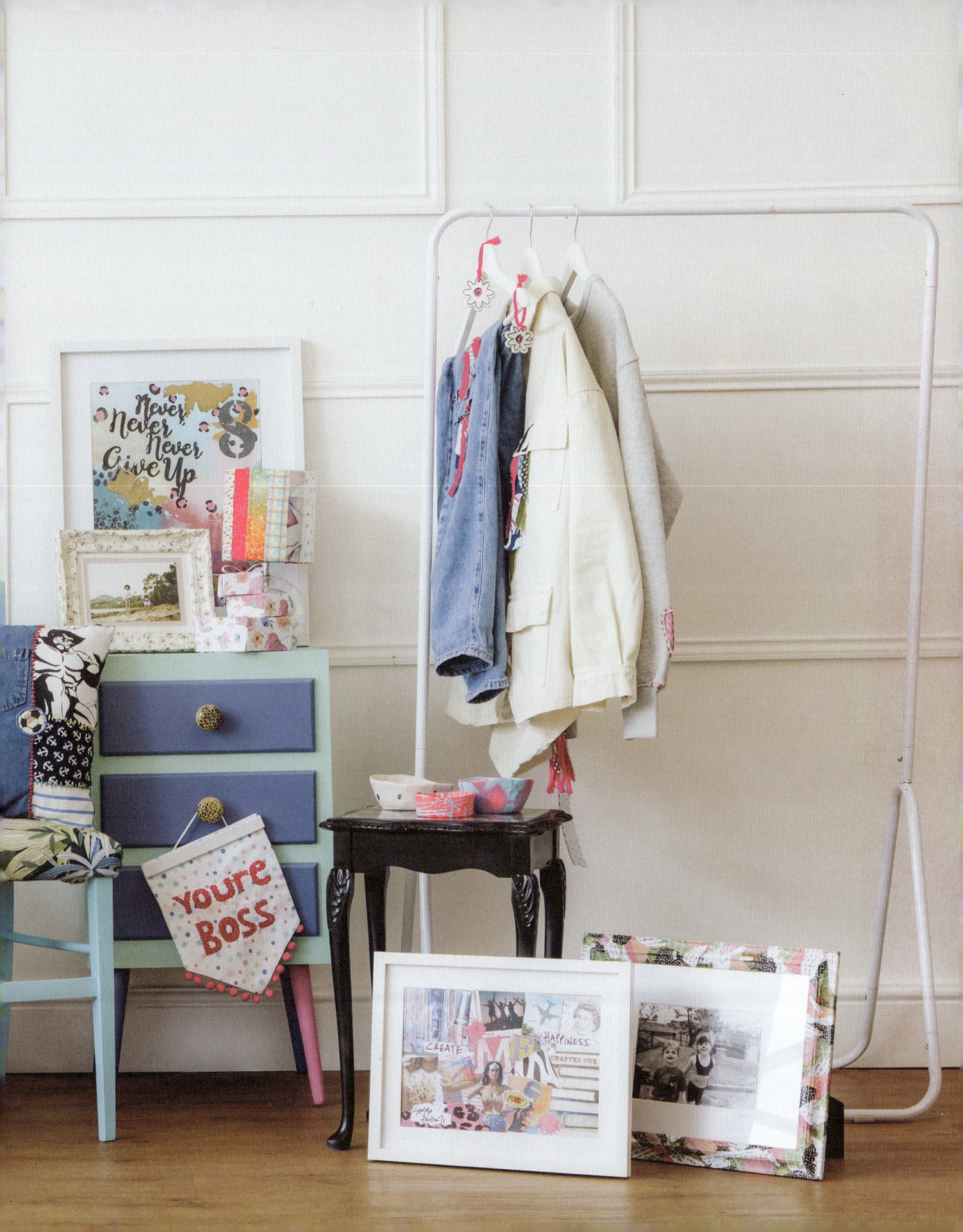

"Gemma's book is a vibrant celebration of the healing power of arts and crafts. Her love of colour shines through every page, showing how immersing yourself in a creative project can really bring a sense of inner calm. A must-read for anyone seeking solace and self-discovery through creativity and fun!"

"This is a joyous and inspirational book for anybody who wants to use creativity to support their wellbeing. Gemma's passion and love of crafting shines through every page and there are loads of brilliant ideas, beautifully presented, to get you started. I loved this book!"

"Gemma's book offers relatable, colourful crafting, approachable for everyone, with picture guides and personal stories paired with art therapy. A stunning and colourful book – great for anyone!"

"Gemma shows us such a fun and pop way of upcycling and recreating our small treasures!"

CRAFT YOUR CURE

25 CRAFT AND UPCYCLING PROJECTS TO HEAL AND BRING JOY

GEMMA LONGWORTH

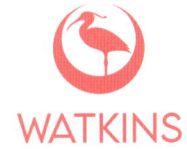

WATKINS

CRAFT YOUR CURE

Gemma Longworth

First published in the UK and USA
in 2025 by Watkins, an imprint of
Watkins Media Limited
Unit 11, Shepperton House,
83–93 Shepperton Road
London N1 3DF

enquiries@watkinspublishing.com

A CIP record for this book is available
from the British Library

ISBN: 978-1-7867-8904-4 (Paperback)
ISBN: 978-1-7867-8905-1 (eBook)

10 9 8 7 6 5 4 3 2 1

Commissioning Editor: Ella Chappell
Managing Editors: Daniel Culver and
    Sophie Blackman
Head of Design: Karen Smith
Cover Design: Alice Claire Coleman
Interior Designers: Alice Claire Coleman
    and Sneha Alexander
Photography: Katrina Lipska –
    Kat's Films
Illustrations: Shutterstock
Production: Uzma Taj

www.watkinspublishing.com

The manufacturer's authorised representative
in the EU for product safety is EU Responsible
Person (for authorities only) – eucomply OÜ –
Pärnu mnt 139b-14, 11317 Tallinn, Estonia,
hello@eucompliancepartner.com,
www.eucompliancepartner.com

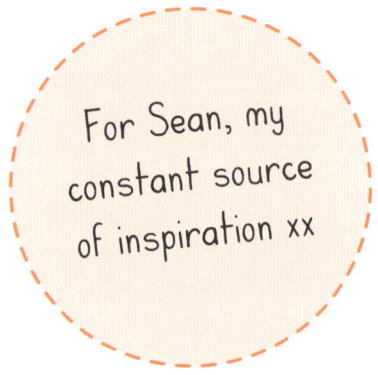

For Sean, my constant source of inspiration xx

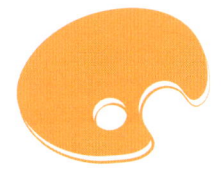 # CONTENTS

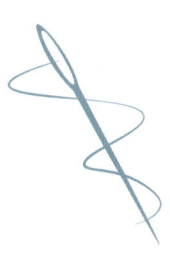

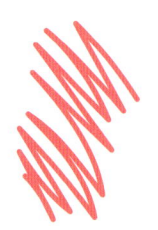

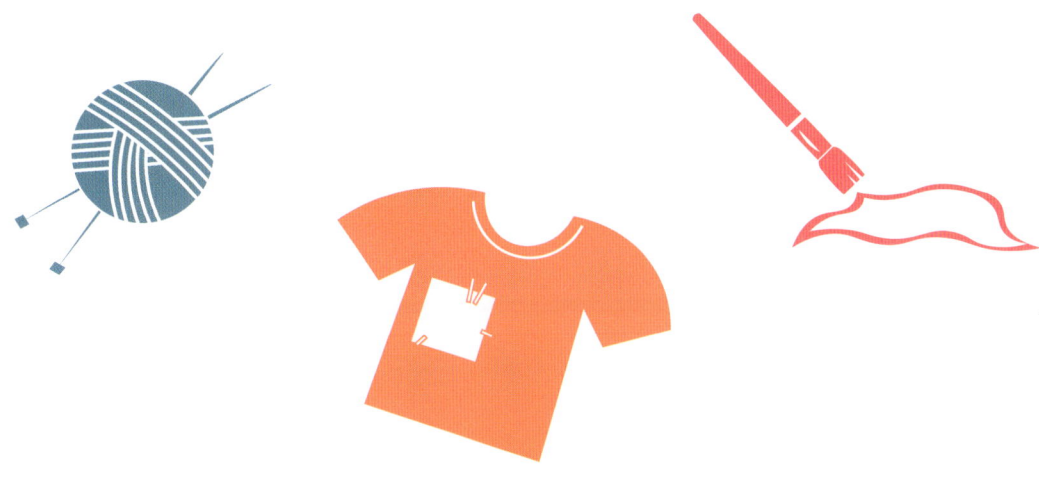

ABOUT THE AUTHOR

Gemma Longworth is an artist, craft expert and TV personality best known as the co-host of *Find It, Fix It, Flog It*, where she shares her love for restoration and upcycling. Growing up as a bereaved sibling, Gemma found solace and healing in art, using creativity as a way to process grief and find resilience. This deeply personal connection to art has fuelled her passion for helping others experience the therapeutic benefits of creativity.

With this mission in mind, Gemma recently founded her own Community Interest Company, Hidden Gems CIC, dedicated to supporting others through creative expression and therapeutic art. Gemma is celebrated for her arts and craft workshops and playful approach to DIY and artisanal restoration. She continues to inspire a wide audience, combining her creative expertise with compassion, encouraging others to see the beauty and potential in both everyday objects and in themselves.

INTRODUCTION

Hi, I'm Gemma, arts and crafts enthusiast and down-to-earth regular northern gal. If you're based in the UK, you may have seen me on the award-winning daytime TV show *Find It, Fix It, Flog It*, upcycling and restoring the nation's unwanted furniture from boring to brilliant. I love working on the show: we have so much fun, plus it gives me the opportunity to demonstrate how transformations can be made through creativity.

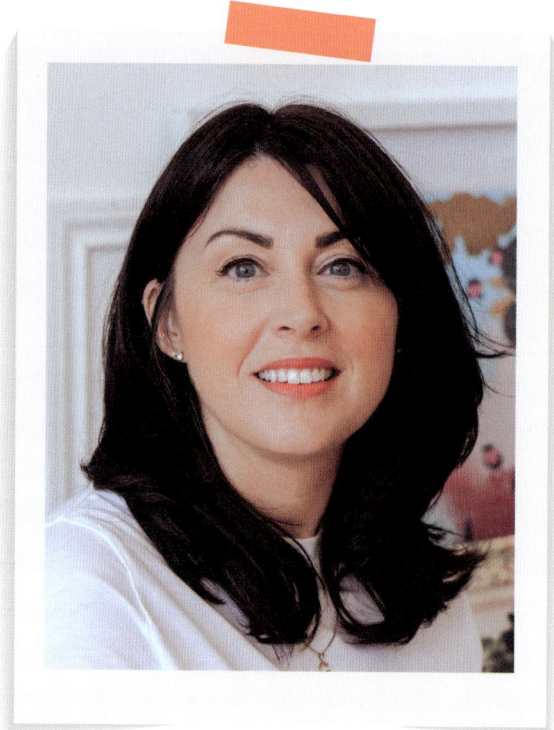

Actually, I'm not just any northerner, I am a scouser, and I feel it's important to mention this, as us scousers are extremely proud. For those that don't know what a scouser is, it's someone who comes from Liverpool, a city here in the UK. A scouser, also known as a Liverpudlian, is generally an all-round awesome person with a brilliant personality, great sense of humour and friendly demeanour!

I have had my own creative business running arts and crafts workshops for the last 20 years, in which I encourage anyone and everyone to be creative and reap the magical benefits the creative process provides us.

Creating is my thing; painting, drawing, sewing, I will try my hand at it all. I've explored art and craft during the many stages of my life, and do you know what? It's really helped me through some very dark times. I appreciate that you may not have much spare time in your extremely busy day, but MAKING a little time for yourself, CREATING some downtime is vital for your mental health.

When my creative journey began

My creative journey began when I was a child. At the age of nine my little brother Sean died. He was in a road accident whilst playing hide and seek outside the family home. Sean was the artist, he would draw constantly, his muse was Sonic the Hedgehog, although this could change on a whim to Dracula or one of the Power Rangers ... never the pink one, though!

Sean and I had the typical brother-and-sister relationship. We annoyed each other, we bickered, he told everyone in school that I had nits, and no one would sit next to me for weeks! As revenge I pulled him off the couch by his legs and his front tooth went through his lip! Oops!

But we loved each other, we were a pair ... Gemma and Sean, Rosie and Jim, Sharky and George. (Sharky and George were an animated crime-fighting duo of the sea in the 1990s that Sean and I loved to watch together.)

I was 11 when Sean died, old enough to know he was never coming back and old enough for my heart to shatter into a million pieces. Not old enough to process all the emotions that came with his loss, though. On 7 August 1996 my life changed for ever. My mum was devastated, my family shattered, my friends felt sorry for

me ... every existing relationship in my life either gone or changed significantly.

I turned to art initially as a way to remember my brother, to keep him with me. I wasn't as good at drawing as Sean, but it wasn't about my abilities or even the finished drawing; it was the process of drawing to keep Sean close. Creating as a way to process emotions has stayed with me; it has shaped who I am today.

Although this tragedy is where my journey began, I do feel I would have somehow found this creative path regardless. I have a passion for creating, doing and making. Putting pen to paper has never come naturally to me – which is ironic really, as I'm now writing a book.

Losing Sean was my first experience of such overwhelming, all-consuming, powerful emotions, emotions that would impact my life dramatically and change who I am. Today, as a 40-year-old woman, I've experienced my fair share of life's challenges, dark times and low moments. I've experienced heartbreaks and losses, depression and anxiety ... the full works! I'm also not naive to think that I don't have more to face.

But during these dark times, creativity has been my light.

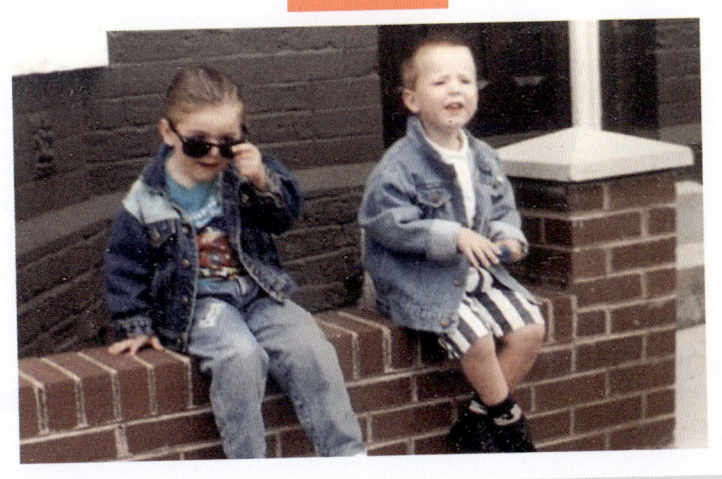

ART AS THERAPY

I started using art as a therapeutic tool when I lost my brother Sean; however, at the time I was unaware that I was using art as a form of therapy. I was a creative kid and loved all things art and crafts. But when I lost Sean, art took on a whole new role; it was my comfort blanket and my safe space.

I was creative to feel close to my brother, to express my emotions, to bring a little joy to my days. Making art and crafting became my passion and my obsession, so of course it was my subject of choice when I left school. It was during my studies that I came across art therapy and realized this is how I had been using art for many years. It was a revelation.

Art therapy is a useful form of psychotherapy that utilizes the creative process of making art to improve mental, emotional and physical wellbeing. It involves the use of various art materials and techniques to help individuals better express themselves, explore their emotions and process difficult experiences. Art therapy is delivered by a trained professional. However, you can still reap the benefits of art through your own creative practice without seeing a licensed psychotherapist, just like I have.

Creating art regularly has proven to help people all over the world overcome trauma, depression, anxiety and stress. Research has shown it can actually improve physical pain too! For many, creating art can be a cathartic outlet for emotional expression and release. Art is a powerful form of expression for those who may find it difficult to verbalize their thoughts, feelings or experiences. Through art-making, you can communicate and explore your inner world in a nonverbal manner.

Producing art and crafting can have a calming and soothing effect on the mind and body, similar to meditation or mindfulness practices. It can help us relax and destress and can improve overall wellbeing. Not only that, it can boost self-esteem and self-confidence, improve communication and social skills and facilitate personal growth and transformation. Through the process of art-making, we can tap into our creativity, resourcefulness and inner strengths to overcome obstacles and thrive.

Completing projects and seeing the results of our efforts can foster a sense of accomplishment.

CREATIVITY

Now, I know what lots of you will be thinking … I'm not creative! I hear it all the time. I agree that some of us are more creative than others, but all of us are creative in our own way.

Creative people are said to be more open to trying new things, will happily play with new ideas, tend to learn from their mistakes and are more likely to take risks and step outside their comfort zone.

In general, creativity is the ability to generate new ideas, concepts or solutions, often through the use of imagination, originality and innovation. Being creative involves thinking outside the box, breaking free from conventional patterns or limitations, and exploring new possibilities.

Creativity shows up in many forms and contexts, from artistic expression through the likes of dance, literature and music to scientific innovation to everyday problem-solving.

My creativity is at home within the visual arts. Through the process of producing art and crafting, I can communicate my thoughts and feelings in a unique way. I find experimenting with a variety of mediums and materials a meaningful visual way to express myself. This creative expression has become part of my identity.

The best way to allow arts and crafts to become part of your identity is to form a creative routine.

A CREATIVE ROUTINE

Like anything in life, you get out of it what you put in; so, to gain the biggest rewards from the process of creating, you need to create. Little and often would be my advice, but it's important you take this at your own pace, so that it isn't a chore.

Producing art and crafts is a process for you to enjoy. If you include it in your daily routine, it will become a healthy habit and you will see results. The more you do the better. Research has shown that creating art for as little as 20 minutes per day can lower your cortisol and reduce stress and symptoms of anxiety.

Coming from someone who struggles to remember to drink one glass of water a day, I can understand that 20 minutes a day of crafting may seem like a lot to begin with, so let's aim for that as a goal.For now, create as often as you can and be accountable for giving yourself this time.

You might want to get up before everyone else to give yourself some time to create, to clear your mind and put yourself in a positive mindset for the rest of the day. Maybe you would prefer to create at night, to unwind and reflect on the day. Or perhaps over lunch would suit you best ... Whenever you have the time, use it wisely, create, make, unwind and thrive.

A SPACE TO CREATE

Where you create can also have an impact on your mindset and overall productivity. The perfect space to craft will be different for everyone. You want an environment that inspires creativity and makes you feel comfortable and motivated.

For most, that's a space in your home that suits your crafting needs and preferences. It could be a spare room, a corner of your living room or even a dedicated area in your bedroom.

I live alone so my entire house is my creative space. I love nothing more than crafting in front of the TV on a winter's night, fire on, candles lit, with a large hot cup of tea. But I also have my spare room, which I have turned into my crafting studio. I work here when I'm feeling more energized or determined, when I mean business.

If you're anything like me, you will want to organize and declutter the space you're working from. If I have too much clutter around me, it distracts me and I find it difficult to focus.

You may want to personalize the space by displaying your artwork, favourite quotes or special photographs that resonate with you.

Essentially, the perfect crafting space is ultimately one that reflects your personality, supports your creative process and makes you feel inspired and empowered to bring your artistic visions to life. So, make yourself comfortable.

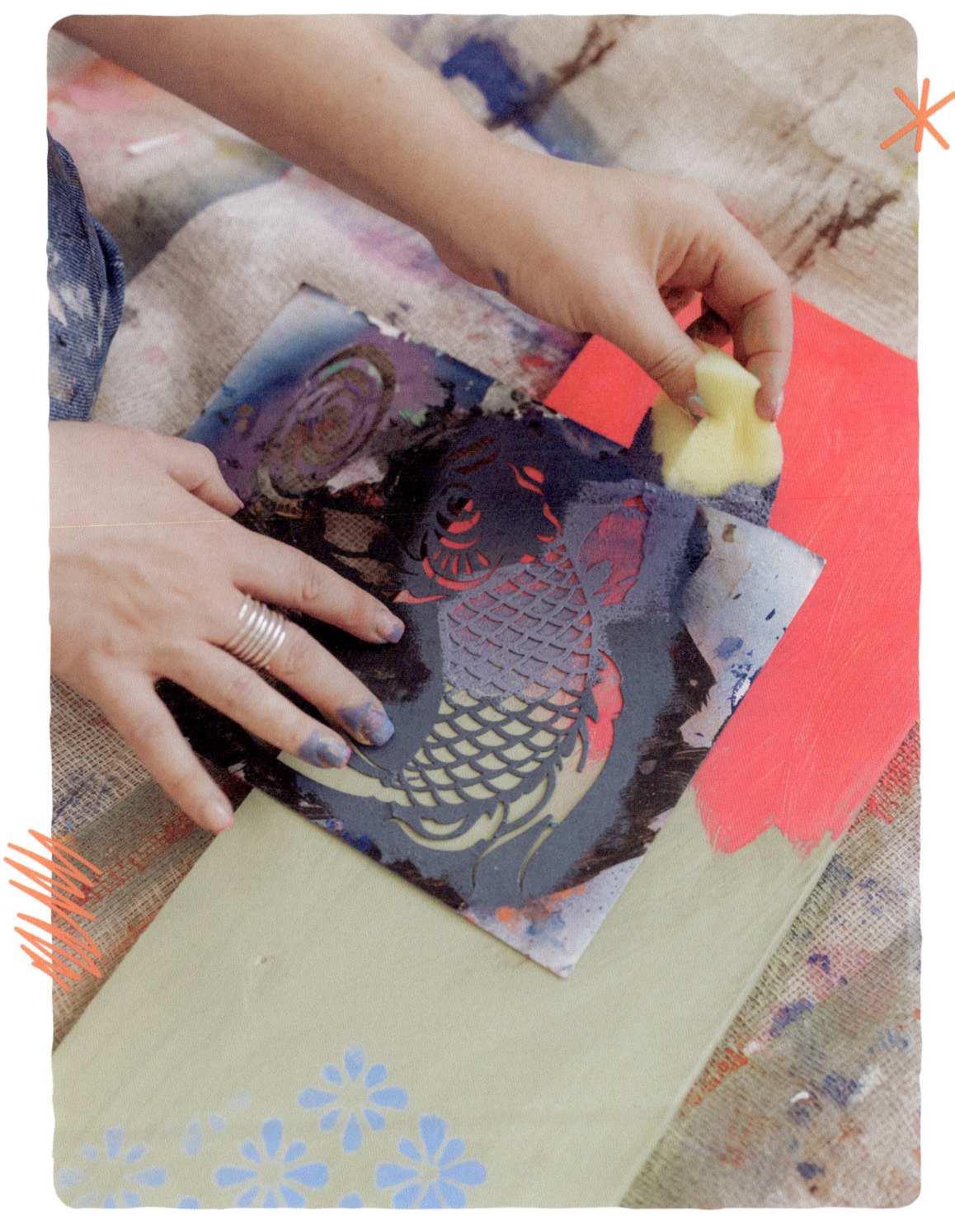

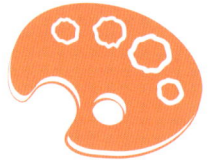

COLOUR

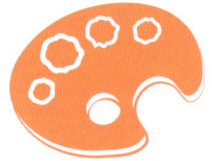

Oh, I love colour! The brighter, bolder, more garish, the better for me. I try to fill my life with as much colour as possible – my home, my wardrobe, my crafts, even my plate.

Bright colours put a smile on my face and certain colours make me feel a certain way. I do have a not-so-secret love affair with the colour pink. For me pink signifies playfulness, confidence and joy. I use it in my crafts as often as I can.

We all subconsciously make emotional connections to colours and are drawn to some more than others. This is something I have explored at length during my art studies. The concept of colour association is something I have to consider when producing artworks for hospitals, when upcycling furniture for interiors and when creating with patients expressing powerful emotions. Certain colours can make or break the mood and it's crucial you get it right in settings such as these.

Colours have a profound effect on our mood and emotions because of their psychological associations and cultural meanings. Therefore, it is important to think about your colour choices when creating your arts and crafts. The

activities in this book encourage you to have some me time, to relax, unwind, express and reflect, and choosing the right colours to lift your mood can enhance the process dramatically.

So have a think about your favourite colours and which ones put a smile on your face. Let's run through the most common associations to help you create your ultimate mood-boosting colour palette …

★ **Red** – Red is often associated with passion, energy and excitement. It can evoke feelings of power, intensity and urgency. However, it can also be associated with aggression or danger in certain contexts.

★ **Orange** – Orange is a warm and energetic colour that can evoke feelings of enthusiasm, creativity and optimism. It's often associated with vitality and warmth, making it a great choice for portraying a sense of comfort.

★ **Yellow** – Yellow is a bright, cheerful colour that is often associated with happiness, positivity and optimism. It can evoke feelings of warmth, energy and hopefulness. However, too much yellow can be overwhelming and may lead to feelings of anxiety or irritability in some individuals.

★ **Green** – Green is a calming and soothing colour that is often associated with nature, growth and renewal. It can evoke feelings of balance, harmony and tranquillity. Green is also associated with health and vitality, making it a good choice for promoting relaxation and for stress relief.

★ **Blue** – Blue is a calming and serene colour that is often associated with peace, stability and trustworthiness. It can evoke feelings of relaxation, clarity and introspection. However, it's important to note that different shades of blue can have varying effects, with lighter shades being more calming and darker shades being more sombre or gloomy.

★ **Purple** – Purple is a rich and luxurious colour that is often associated with creativity, spirituality and wisdom. It can evoke feelings of mystery, introspection and inspiration. Purple is also associated with royalty and sophistication, making it a good choice for promoting a sense of luxury and elegance.

★ **Pink** – Pink is a gentle and nurturing colour that is often associated with love, compassion and femininity. It can evoke feelings of warmth, affection and tenderness. Pink is also associated with innocence and playfulness, making it a good choice for promoting a sense of comfort and nurturing.

★ **Neutral colours** – Neutral colours such as white, grey and beige evoke feelings of balance and calmness. They can provide a sense of simplicity, grounding and stability, making them a good choice for creating a peaceful and harmonious environment.

⊕ It's important to remember that individual experiences with colour can vary based on personal preferences, cultural background and past experiences. Additionally, different combinations of colours can have unique effects on mood, so consider how different colours interact with each other when creating your works of art and crafts.

This may seem like a lot to consider, but the bottom line is use what colours make you happy and express your mood. No need to overthink it. I'm sure you will notice a running colour theme throughout this book ... all my personal favourites.

Live your life in full colour; it's a much more fun and vibrant place.

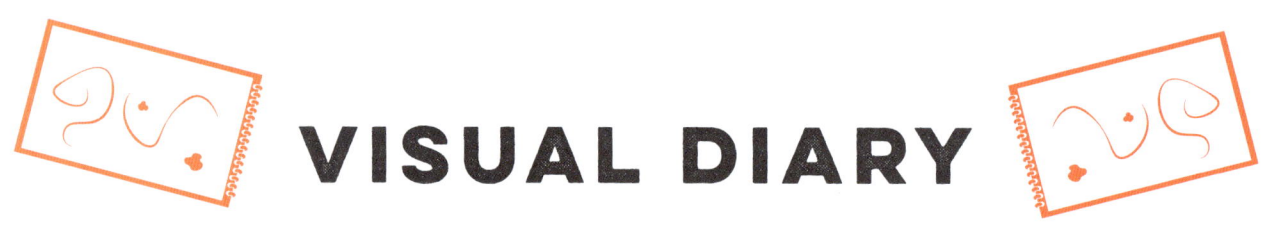

VISUAL DIARY

A visual diary, also known as an art journal or sketchbook, is a personal creative project where you can express your thoughts and your emotions visually through a combination of artistic mediums and techniques. A visual diary is just like a written diary in that it's a reflection of you, but the focus is on the images rather than words.

To truly reap the powerful positive benefits of the creative process, you need to be creating regularly. Like anything, the more you put in the more you get out. Now, of course we can't be creating a masterpiece every day, not even Van Gogh did that, but creating little and often will keep our creative muscle growing. The aim is to create a healthy habit that allows us to blossom.

Many years ago when I was at university studying art and design, I was encouraged to use a visual diary by my tutors. As a part of the course, you would show your research, ideas, experiments and reflections in the form of a visual diary. This is something that has stuck with me since graduating and has been incredibly beneficial to me in many ways.

THE BENEFITS OF A VISUAL DIARY

Now, I'm fortunate to work within the creative industry, so I'm taking part in arts, crafts and DIY projects daily, and I like to think this is keeping my creative brain ticking over. But I do still use my visual diary regularly. I tend to work on one sketchbook at a time, gathering ideas and creating smaller pieces of artwork when I don't have the time or need to create something larger. When one diary is full I always keep it for reference and inspiration. They are such lovely things to look back on. My visual diary keeps my creativity flowing. I use mine every day and here's why I think you should too:

★ **Therapeutic benefits** – Visual diaries can help to reduce stress, help us cope with difficult emotions, increase self-awareness and encourage self-compassion. They are often used as a form of therapy in clinical settings, as they can have therapeutic benefits for mental health and wellbeing.

★ **Personal expression** – My visual diary is very personal. It reflects my thoughts, feelings, experiences and interests. It reads like a story of my life and experiences and provides me with a safe and non-judgemental space for self-expression. It can help me to process my emotions.

★ **Reflection and insight** – My visual diary is a tool for self-reflection. Through the act of creating and reflecting on my work, I can gain insight into my thoughts, emotions and experiences, and this reflection can often leave me with a new perspective on difficult situations.

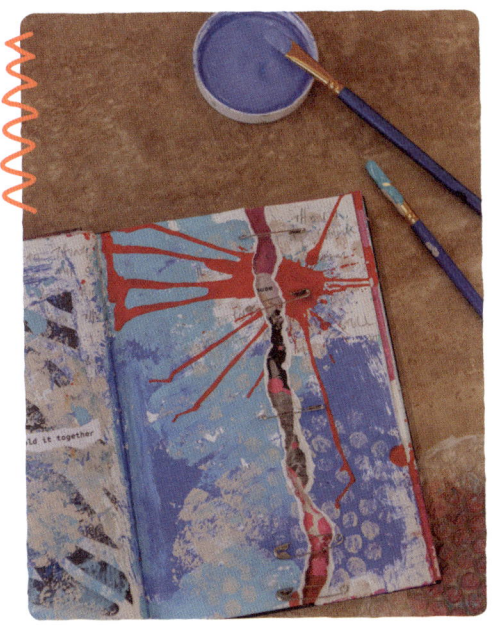

★ **New mediums** – My visual diaries often include a variety of techniques and materials. I try out different drawing and painting styles, collage, photography and, on occasions when the mood strikes me, poetry. This use of mixed media allows me to explore creative techniques, which often leads to inspiration for my other art and craft projects.

★ **The creative process** – My visual diary allows me to embrace the process over the end result. It's a way to engage with the creative process in a spontaneous, intuitive and playful manner. You are not working toward an end goal, so there are no rules or expectations. You can make mistakes and move on.

★ **Keeping memories** – Visual diaries also serve as a record of daily life, special occasions and memorable experiences. They can capture memories, moments and events, as well as document personal growth and transformation over time.

Getting started

A visual diary gets you in a routine of creating daily. It is an exciting habit that sparks inspiration for larger projects. Remember that your visual journal is a personal and evolving journey, so feel

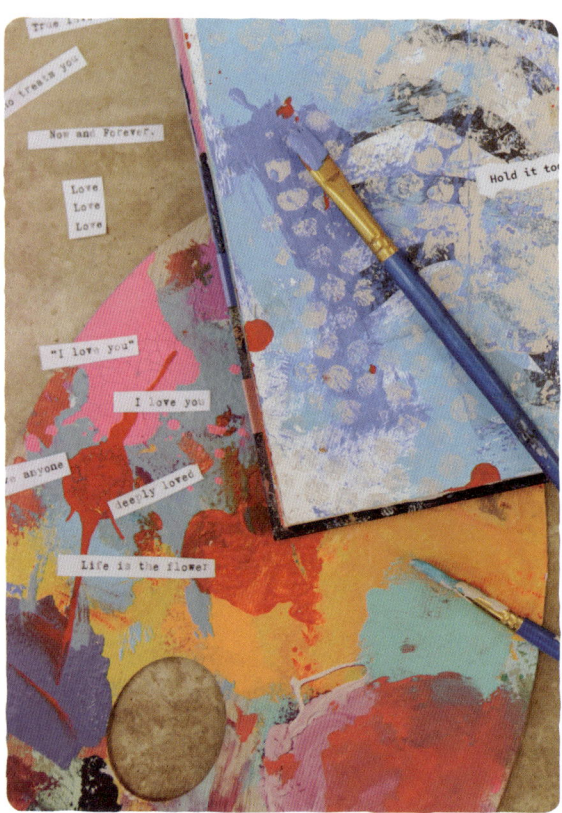

From a quick doodle while you're anxiously waiting at the doctor's, to absent-minded line-making when you're sitting relaxed on the beach on your jollies, there is always time to create.

Over time your visual diary will become something meaningful to you and something you will truly enjoy creating.

A few ideas to get you started

Collage with collected images and cutouts from magazines — for example, images of artworks that inspire you, with notes on what you love about these particular pieces.

Drawing quick, simple daily sketches — I like to draw items that surround me, from my bedside lamp, my coffee and biscuits to the flowers in my garden.

Painting, playing with mark-making or colour compositions — watercolour painting is great for florals and landscapes.

free to experiment, explore and make it your own. Allow yourself the freedom to create without judgement and enjoy the process of self-expression and discovery.

There is no materials list for a visual diary, as it is personal to each individual. So, if you draw you will need a pen/pencil, if you paint you will need paints and a brush ... it really is up to you.

I like to work with sketchbooks, but you could always collate your work in a folder. I use a smaller sketchbook, as I find it's more practical for carrying around with me and I can have it on hand for whenever the mood strikes me.

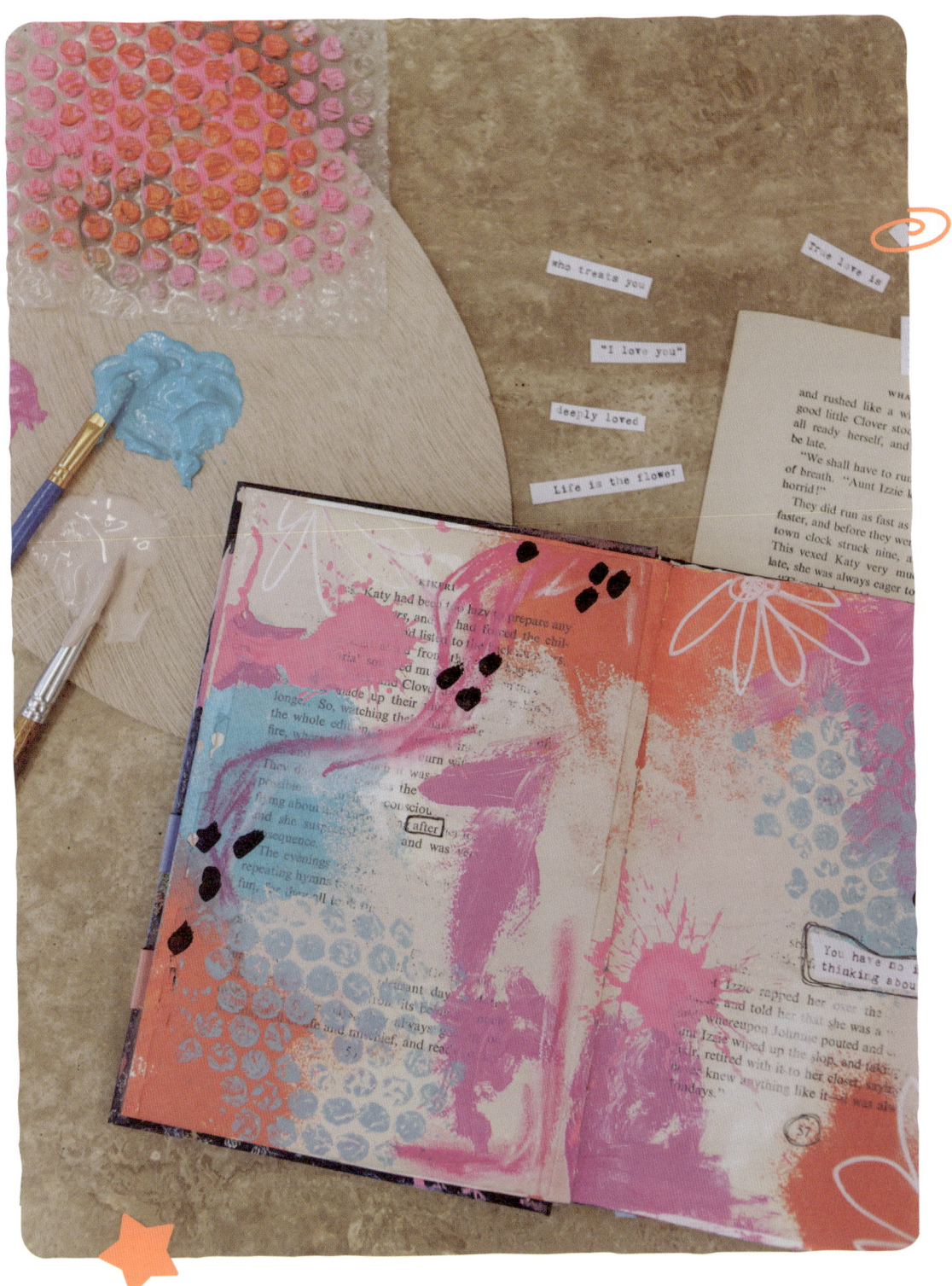

VISION BOARDS

A vision board is a crafting activity for creatively visualizing your goals, wants and needs. This activity requires thought and self-reflection, and therefore it's a good starting point for using crafts as a mindfulness tool.

A vision board is a visual representation of your goals, dreams and aspirations. It typically consists of images, words and other visual elements that represent the things you want to achieve or manifest for your life. Creating a vision board can help you to clarify your goals, visualize your desired future and stay focused and on the right path to achieving it.

When we focus on working toward our goals, we feel more confident, stronger and able. When we have clear goals, we can make decisions more easily and problem solve more effectively.

I've never been too good with words, and putting pen to paper or keeping a written diary just doesn't appeal to me. So, for me, a vision board is a great

way to get thoughts and ideas out of my head and down on paper. I find this frees up a little space in my mind. Believe me, it's cluttered up there. I'm like a thought hoarder, a massive overthinker!

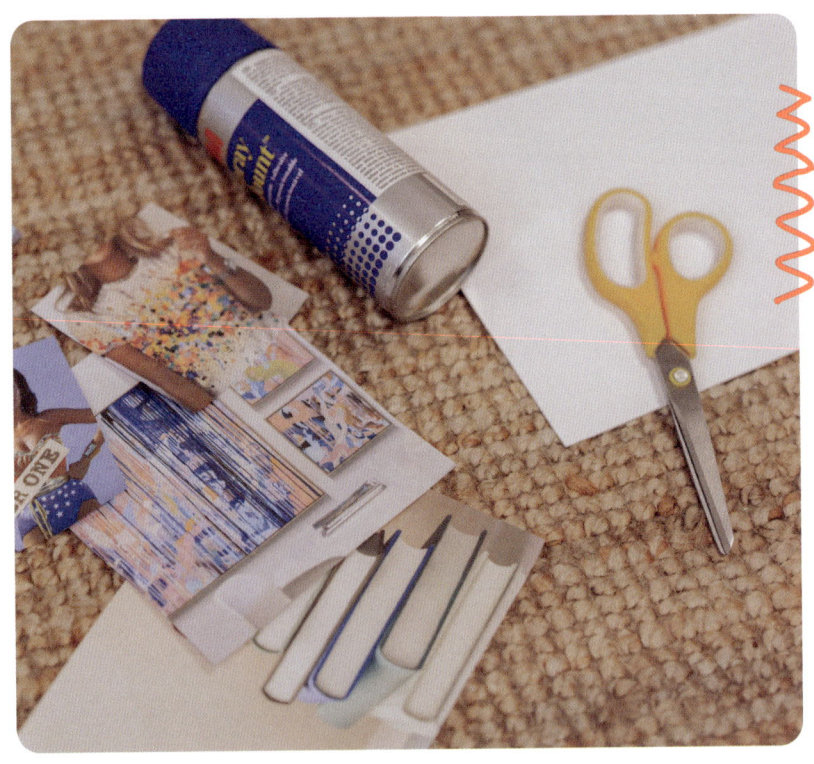

My first vision board

We all have goals and dreams for our future. When we are young, we dream BIG, and nothing seems off limits. As we get older, reality kicks in and our expectations become a little lower. When I was a child, I wanted to be a fashion designer. From the age of six or seven, I dreamed of everyone wearing my colourful creations ... I would walk down the runway while everyone clapped, and I would spend my days wearing huge sunglasses and eating cupcakes (that's what fashion designers do, of course!). I would be so sophisticated!

With that in mind, I spent most of my time on my fashion wheel, creating endless combinations of outfits. For those of you that haven't seen a fashion wheel, it was a popular toy in the 1990s, a layered wheel of items of clothing which you turned to create different outfit combinations. I kept all my designs in my blue folder, which I carried at all times. Looking back, this was almost like my first ever vision board.

This dream stuck with me for a while, and I eventually enrolled for a degree in fashion and textiles. I soon realized that fashion wasn't for me, so I focused on the textiles element of the course. It felt more personally expressive and less about the consumer. It was during my textiles studies that I began to explore a connection between fabric and comfort, and this eventually led me to create for my own comfort. I realized I had been using art to heal from my traumas for all these years. This discovery opened my eyes to a whole world of art as therapy.

When to do a vision board

One of the best times to create a vision board is at the beginning of the year, to plan and manifest your goals for the year ahead, both personal and professional. I like to do it more often, twice or even three times a year. A vision board affirms my plans and helps me stay motivated and on track. It has become a great tool for gaining clarity when my mind starts to run away with itself, which it often does.

It was while I was studying for my master's in textiles that I discovered I was dyslexic. When I was writing my dissertation I realized I was struggling more than most people. I was tested for dyslexia, and it was confirmed. Things began to make sense and although writing is still a struggle for me, I do try to put less pressure on myself when I do have to write ... like now! Often when it comes to writing, I seem to have a mental block. I get distracted by everything, and I mean EVERYTHING. But ask me to create you a vision board, find you some images or paint you a picture, and it's done in a matter of minutes.

CREATING A VISION BOARD

YOU WILL NEED

★ **Cardboard or corkboard** – this will be the base for your vision board. Choose a size that suits your preferences and the space where you will be displaying your board.

★ **Magazines, newspapers and images** – you can buy vision board books that come with lots of images that you might need for your board, but I personally love the process of scouring through magazines to find what resonates with me.

★ **Scissors**

★ **Glue or tape** – you can use glue sticks, PVA glue, double-sided tape

or even drawing pins if you've opted for a corkboard base.

★ **Markers or pens** – you may want to add affirmations, goals or additional words by writing them directly onto the board. I like to add wording in my own handwriting to make it more personal.

★ **Embellishments (optional)** – you might want to include embellishments such as stickers, ribbons, glitter or other decorative elements to enhance your vision board.

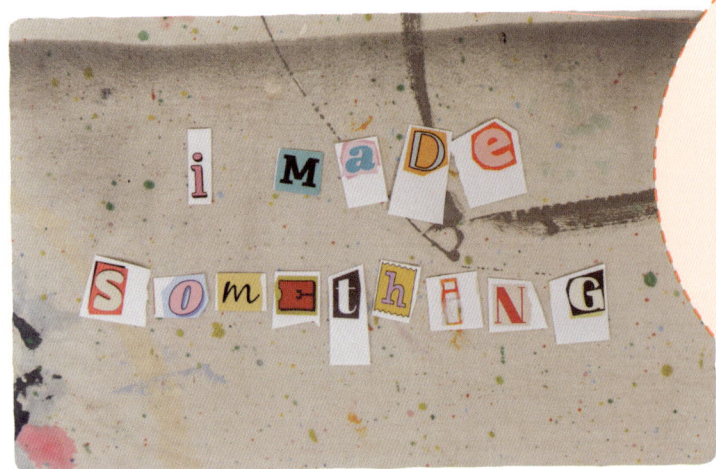

REMEMBER:
that the materials you choose can vary based on your personal preferences and the specific vision you have for your board. The key is to select items that resonate with you and visually represent your goals and aspirations.

HOW TO CREATE A VISION BOARD

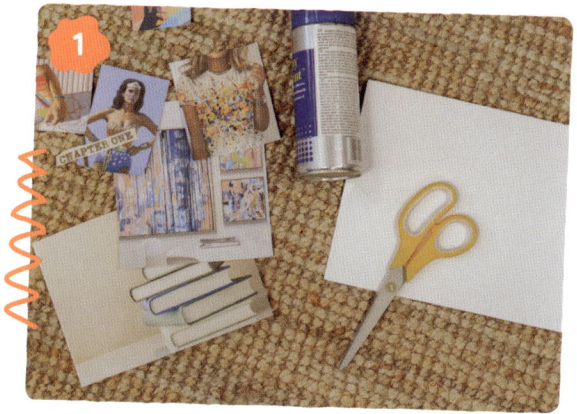

1. The first and most important task at hand is taking the time to gather your thoughts. This requires some YOU time. Find a quiet and comfortable space where you can focus and get creative without distractions. Play some calming music, light a candle or incorporate any other elements that help you feel relaxed and inspired.

2. Try to visualize your goals. Close your eyes if it helps and visualize yourself already achieving your goals. Imagine how you would feel, what you would see, and what your life would look like once you've accomplished them. Use this visualization as inspiration for selecting images and words for your vision board.

The things I want to include on my board

Drink more water

Write a book

Build confidence

Work on friendships

Have more work – life balance

Work toward financial security

Develop personal creativity

Public speaking/presenting

Develop a product

Have more ME time

3. Flick through magazines or search online for images, words and phrases that resonate with your goals and aspirations. Cut or print out the ones that speak to you and represent what you want to manifest in your life.

4. Arrange your images and text on your board. Play around with different layouts until you find a composition that feels right to you. You can organize them by theme, by category, or in any way that makes sense for you.

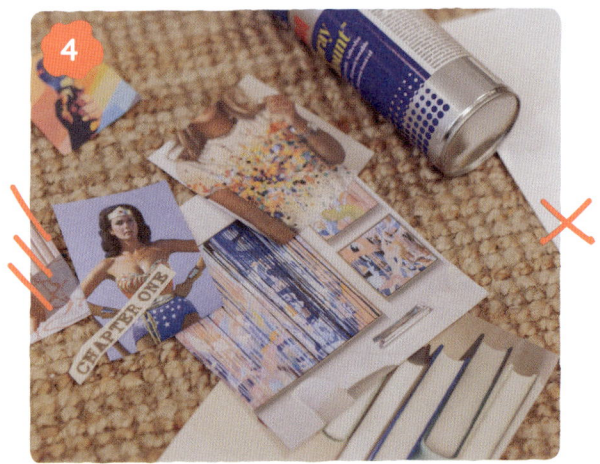

5. Once you're happy with the layout, start gluing or taping the images and words onto the board. Take your time and be mindful as you attach each element, focusing on the intentions behind them.

6. Add personal touches: use markers or pens to write affirmations, goals or additional words directly onto the board. You may wish to include some extra embellishments such as stickers, ribbons or glitter to make your vision board more visually appealing.

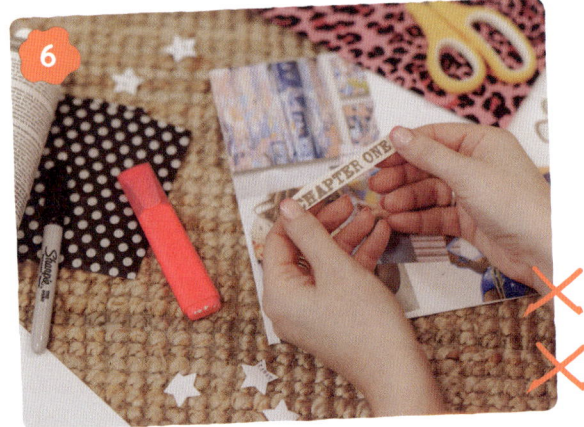

7. Once it's complete, review and reflect. Step back and take a moment to study your vision board. Focus on the images, words and intentions you've chosen, and how they make you feel. Connect with the sense of empowerment and inspiration that comes from visualizing your dreams.

8. Display your vision board: find a prominent place to display it where you'll see it every day – your bedroom wall, office or any other space where you spend a lot of time. Make sure it's easily visible so you can be reminded of your goals and stay focused on manifesting them.

⊕ Remember that your vision board is a personal reflection of YOUR dreams and aspirations. Update it regularly as your goals evolve and new aspirations emerge. Allow yourself to be excited and positive for the future you have planned for yourself. You deserve to be happy.

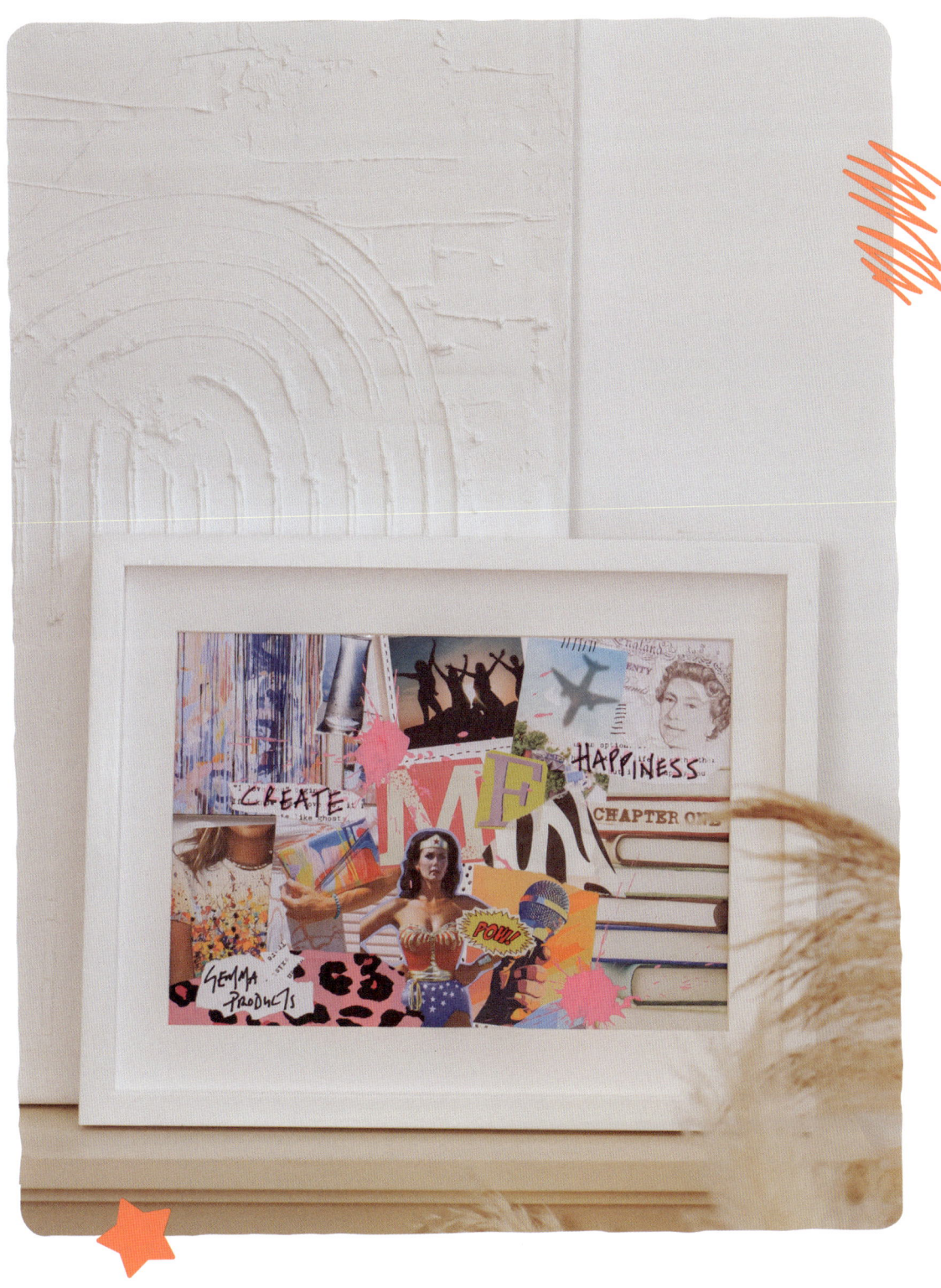

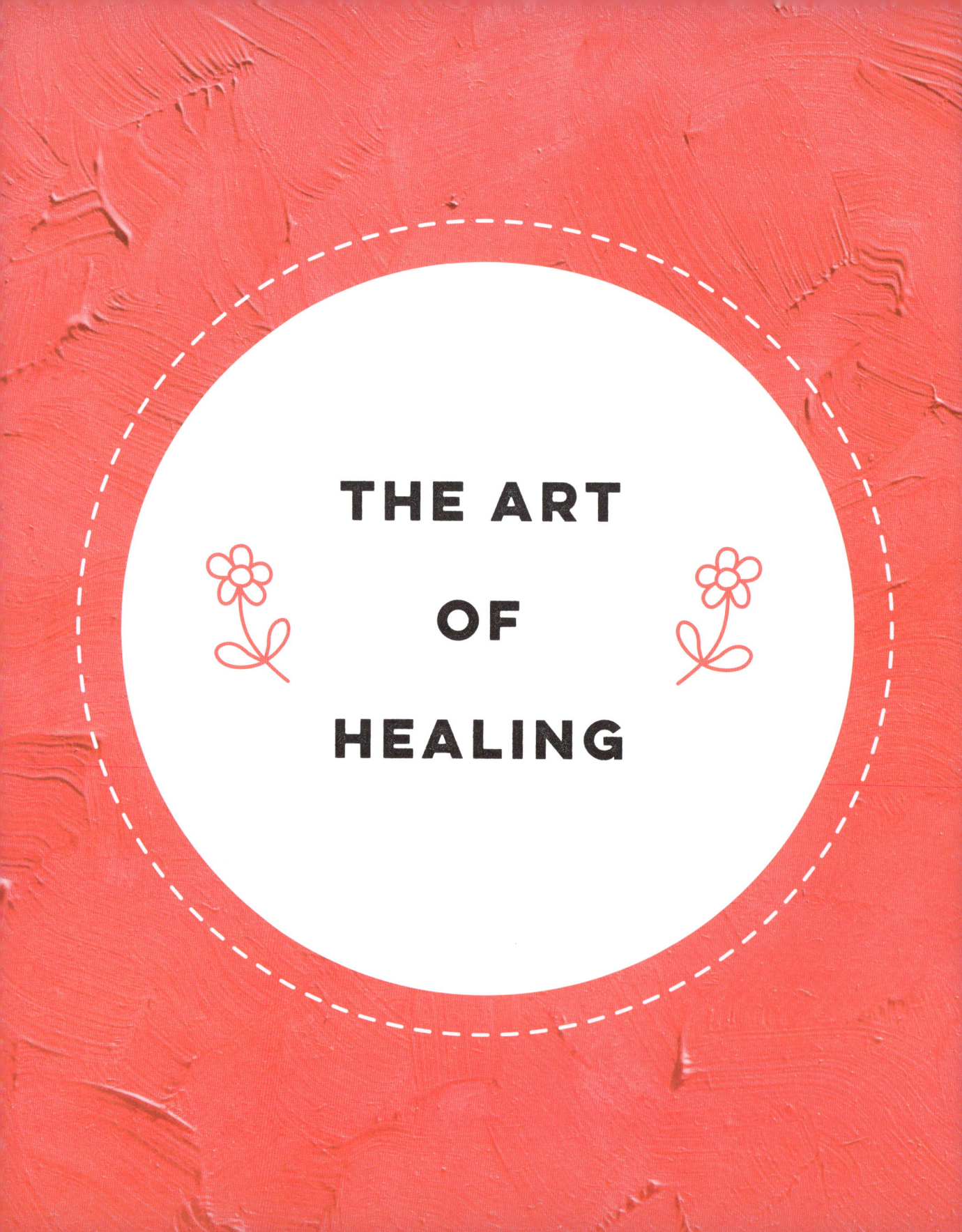

THE ART

OF

HEALING

Looking after our mental health is now more important than ever. Reportedly 1 in 8 people globally are affected by mental health disorders, with anxiety and depression the most common conditions. Depression affects more than 264 million people across the world of all ages – and I'm one of them.

Creating this book has forced me to look at my own mental health and hold up a mirror to the complex individual that is me.

I share these stories with you in the hope that you may relate to something I have experienced. I've been through a lot and I know I'm not alone. Life can be tough, but it's also beautiful. Sometimes the beauty is hard to see, so it's important we look for it.

"... find things beautiful as much as you can, most people find too little beautiful."

– Vincent Van Gogh to his brother Theo, 1874

Art fills my days with beauty. For me, art can be a mindfulness activity that allows me to relax, unwind and give my mind the space it needs to heal. It provides me with a release, an escape, a way of expressing my emotions.

I love to paint and I thrive off upcycling. I'm always on the lookout for new things. In this section I have given you a variety of activities to try so you can hopefully find your own healing practices.

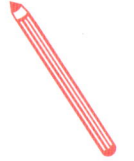

THE PROCESS OF DRAWING

Drawing is a powerful mindfulness tool. The process of drawing allows us to focus and be in the present moment. It's incredibly calming for our mind and creates a sense of relaxation and wellbeing, regardless of the accuracy of the drawing itself.

Sean loved to draw; it was his favourite thing to do. His love of drawing is the reason why I do what I do and the reason why I'm writing this book.

I rememeber he used to replace the sleeves of our VHS tapes with his drawn versions. I still have the version of the *Pretty Woman* movie poster which he drew for me. *Pretty Woman* has always been a favourite of mine.

Growing up we spent a lot of time at our grandparents' house. My grandad is an artist, and he would spend hours drawing with us. We would ask him to draw all sorts of things and were amazed by what he could do. He would sit in his chair with my brother perched on the arm and they would draw everything, from clowns and dinosaurs to the Ninja Turtles.

When we lost Sean, drawing became my way to be close to him, to remember

him and keep his memory alive.

Fashion illustrations became my thing – which sounds so much more impressive than it was! I liked to draw outfits; I would copy them out of magazines and my mum's *Littlewoods* catalogues, changing the colours and patterns to create my own collections. This process of drawing to be close to Sean was the start of my creative journey.

Life drawing

Nowadays, drawing is something I dip in and out of. I usually draw in the planning stages of a project. I sketch my plans for upcycles even if it's only me that is able to decipher them. It helps me to see my designs and ideas on paper. It's easy to make changes at this stage, so these drawings are always super helpful when preparing for a big project.

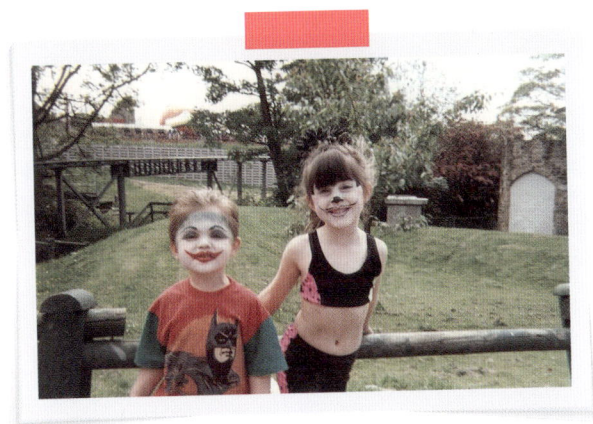

I used to do a lot of life drawing. Life drawing is the practice of drawing the human form, typically the study of a nude model in various poses. The first life drawing class I attended was in art college when I was 18 years old. As you can imagine, the first time there was a bit of blushing and a lot of giggling, but I got over that pretty quickly. We would draw a variety of models, all with different body shapes, but my favourite was Sue Lee, a beautiful curvaceous lady who took life modelling very seriously. She had lots of props – umbrellas, fans and boas, scarves and silks – that she would drape over her body and tie in her hair. My drawings never did her beauty justice, but I always enjoyed the process and often got lost marking out her curves. I found it such a mindful process and I truly felt present in that moment.

I've always been a big fan of colour, so I tried to incorporate colour into my life drawings as often as I could. When others in the class were using charcoal to make their marks, I opted for the brightest oil pastels I could find – red, pinks and oranges – to capture the fierce glamour of Sue Lee. She was never a washed-out pastel pink; she was a bright, bold fuschia.

I recently returned to life drawing when I attended a life drawing social here in Liverpool. It's a rather popular activity nowadays and lots of fun. As I'm usually the one hosting the workshops, it's a real treat for me to attend something like this. Art classes and workshops are great ways to meet people. There's generally a real mixed bag of people, all ages and abilities and from all walks of life. That's what's great about art: it brings people together.

I find being in a workshop environment a great confidence boost because you realize you aren't as bad as you think you are. Actually, you're better than you think you are. There is always someone keen to point out the beauty in your work, even if you can't see it yourself. We must remember it's the process in which we find the most benefit, so don't put pressure on yourself to draw a perfect likeness.

I love to draw in my visual diary, quick doodles that often represent nothing at all. Patterns that grow organically in the moment. Doodling is a great mindfulness activity and something we can do without overthinking it, making it perfect for drawing beginners. If you've ever found yourself scribbling away while on the telephone, this is for you.

DAILY DOODLES

We are going to start off with simple drawing tasks. We will create our own still life, an arrangement of objects that form a composition. Now, we aren't expecting a masterpiece here, we just want to open ourselves up to the process of mindful drawing. Remember that the goal is not to create a perfect or finished artwork, but to engage fully in the process and cultivate awareness of the present moment.

Traditionally a still life consists of things like fruit and flowers, but our arrangement will be made up of objects that say something about us. Choosing items that vary in colour, texture and scale will make for a more interesting composition.

I have three quick observation drawing exercises for you to try with your still life. These activities are just like stretches before running or exercising; they help to loosen us up – because when it comes to drawing, many of us draw the image that's in our minds rather than what's actually in front of us.

These exercises will encourage us to be more playful and expressive and explore different styles of drawing.

Whenever I take the time to draw, I always do at least one of these exercises or all three before doing your stretches before a big run. It really helps me get in the zone. They are fun, simple activities that are great for all the family, for all ages and abilities.

Approach your drawing practice with curiosity, openness and non-judgement, allowing yourself to embrace the experience as it unfolds.

YOU WILL NEED

★ **Something to draw** – gather a selection of items that mean something to you; four or five items will work for now. I'm going for a plant, spotty mug, a selection of colourful threads and my favourite dog ornament.

★ **Something to draw with** – pencil, pen

★ **Something to draw on** – paper, sketchbook

★ **Clock** or **timer**

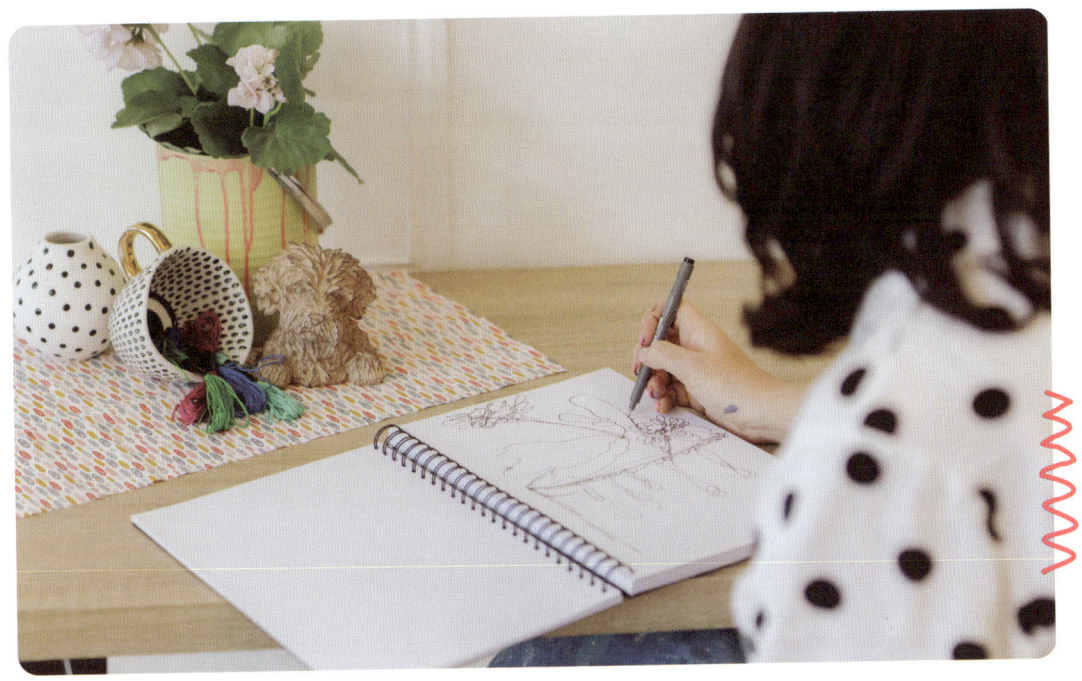

HOW TO DOODLE

1. Arrange your items, thinking about the composition. Make them look appealing, this isn't a line-up. Ideally choose a place where you can leave them for a few days. You may wish to come back to them and draw them again.

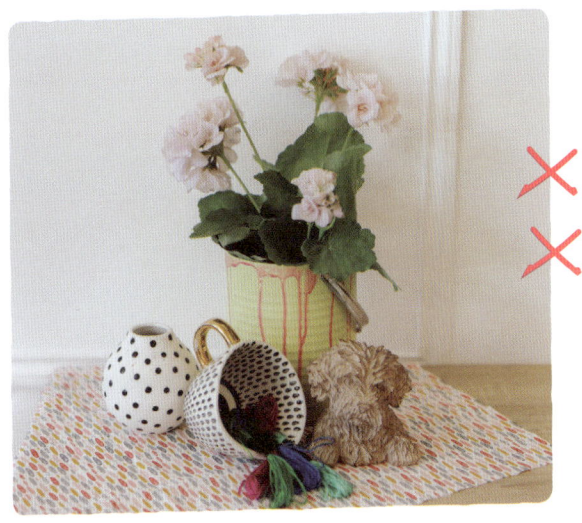

EXERCISE 1: CONTINUOUS LINE

1. Draw what's in front of you without taking your pen/pencil off the page. What we are aiming for is one unbroken continuous line that makes up the entire image. This exercise allows you to capture the composition in its simplest form and creates drawings that often have a unique and spontaneous style.

2. Draw the composition using one continuous line for 5 minutes, then stop.

EXERCISE 2: DRAWING WITH YOUR NON-DOMINANT HAND

1. If you're right-handed, switch to your left, and left-handers switch to your right. You can take your hand off the page this time, but you can only draw using your non-dominant hand. This exercise is a good way to stimulate your creativity and break artistic routines and habits, forcing you to approach your drawing from a different perspective. It often produces unexpected and interesting outcomes. This one is guaranteed to make you smile.

2. Draw the composition using this technique for 5 minutes, then stop.

EXERCISE 3: BLIND CONTOUR DRAWING

1. Blind contour drawing is where you can only look at the composition in front of you and not the drawing. It encourages you to truly look at the composition, improving your observation skills and hand–eye coordination. This is a great one for improving our drawing skills and the ability to see and interpret shapes and proportions accurately. This exercise often produces expressive sketches that capture the essence of the composition rather than the exact details.

2. Draw the composition using this technique for 5 minutes, then stop.

You will now have three drawings of the same composition using three different warm-up techniques. I love to sit mine next to each other and compare. Which one is my favourite? I have also been known to frame mine because everything looks good in a frame!

You can use these exercises to draw anything and everything. They are ideal for workshops and group settings. Drawing each other is always good fun and you're guaranteed to produce some fantastic pieces of art.

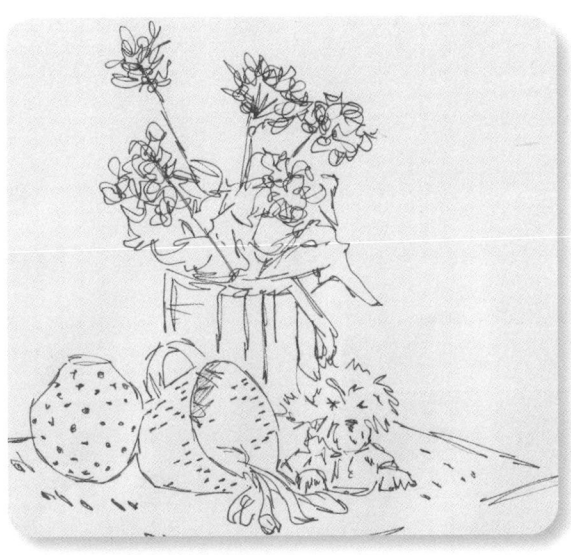

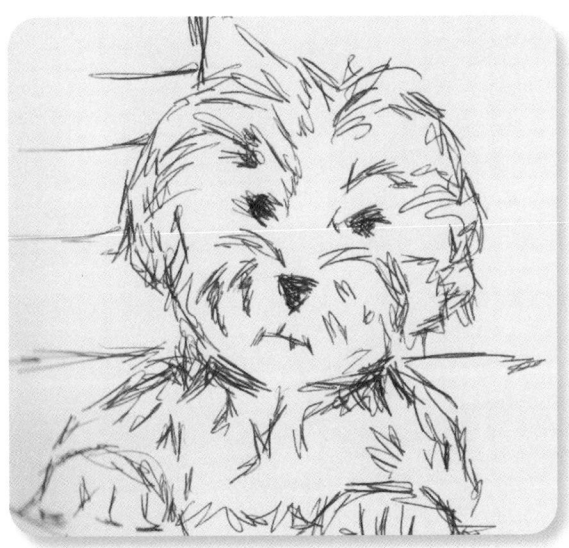

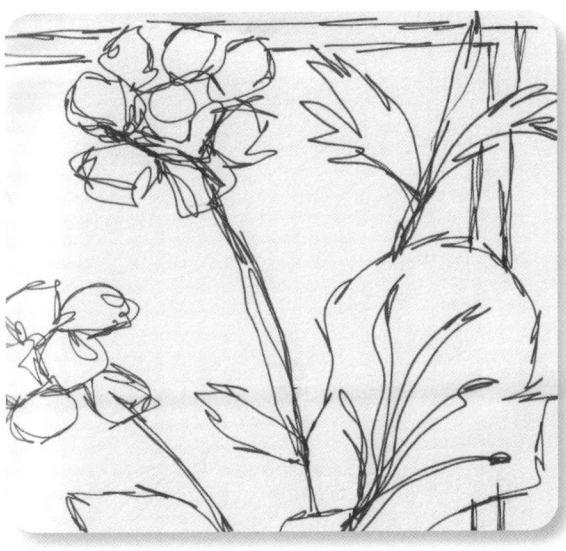

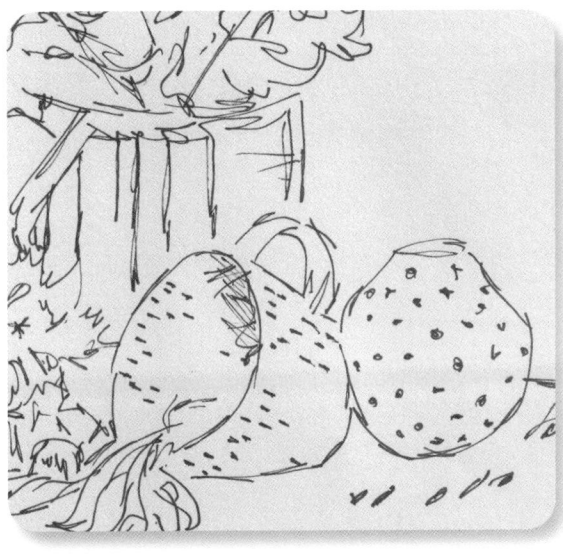

A few more drawing activities

There are many different drawing styles and techniques. If you enjoyed the activities above, here's a few more for you to look into:

★ **Mindful doodling** – Doodling can be a form of spontaneous drawing that allows your mind to wander freely. Set aside a few minutes each day to doodle without any specific goal or plan. Let your pen or pencil move intuitively across the page, exploring shapes, patterns and lines as they emerge.

★ **Zentangle** – Zentangle is a method of drawing structured patterns and designs in a repetitive and meditative manner. Start with a small square piece of paper and draw a simple border around the edges. Then fill the inside with intricate patterns, one small section at a time. Focus on each stroke as you create your design.

★ **Mandala drawing** – Mandala drawing involves creating symmetrical and intricate designs within a circular shape. Start by drawing a circle on your paper as the foundation of your mandala. Then add geometric shapes, lines and patterns radiating outward from the centre. Mandala drawing can be a calming and centring practice.

★ **Nature drawing** – Take your drawing materials outdoors and connect with nature through art. Find a quiet spot, such as a park, garden or forest, and choose a natural subject to draw, such as a tree, flower or rock. Allow yourself to immerse in the sights, sounds and sensations of the natural world as you draw.

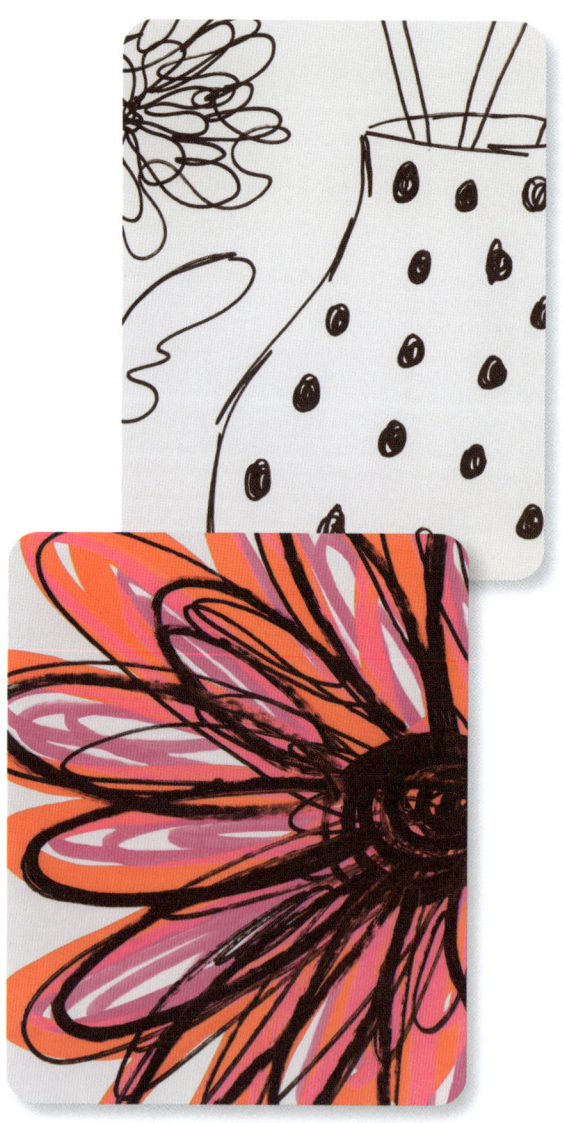

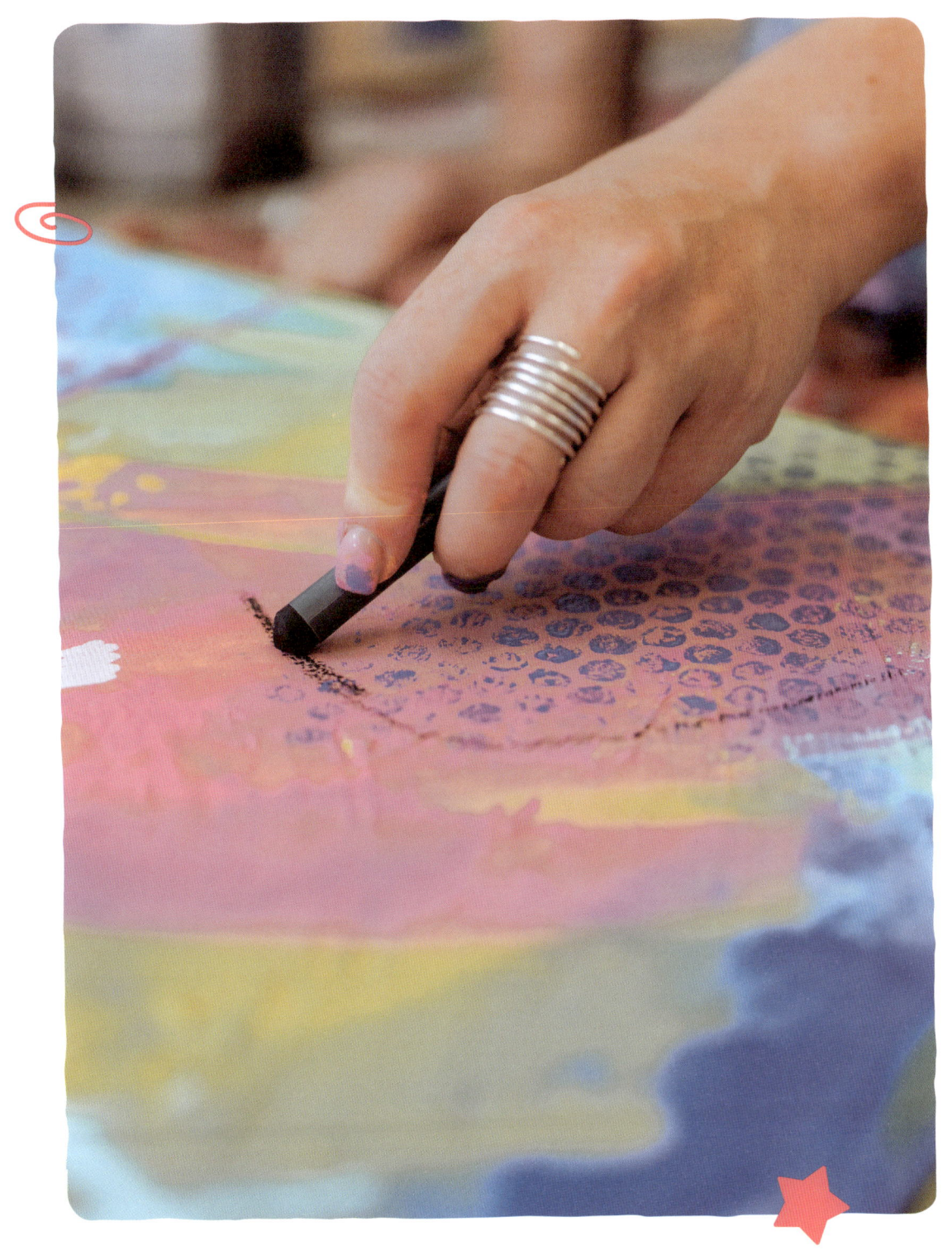

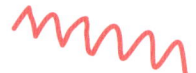

PERSONAL REFLECTION

I think it's crucial that we keep checking in on ourselves, reflecting on who we are and what we want, to allow for personal growth and to strengthen our emotional wellbeing. Take a long, hard look at yourself! Arts and crafts in general are perfect for allowing our minds the time to do just that. The art of self-portraits, however, allows you to focus on you and you alone. Every mark made is a reflection of you.

I live in a three-bedroom terraced house alone. Ok, not completely alone. I do have two guinea pigs called Val and Irene and a goldfish called Vivienne, but I do not count them as company because they are not very sociable.

If I'm honest, I never really wanted guinea pigs. I want a dog. I have mourned for Deirdre, my ginger cavapoo, since the break-up from a previous relationship. He took Deirdre with him when he left. I really loved that dog. A year later I met my current partner, who has curly ginger hair … I do wonder if he's my Deirdre rebound?!

Motherhood

I'm the type of neighbour who likes to keep myself to myself. I'm not one for talking on the step or knocking on their door to borrow a cup of sugar (I've seen this in films and I'm not actually sure if people do it in real life!), but I will take in a parcel if it's required. Honestly, I don't think my neighbours even know my name and I don't know all of theirs.

My next-door neighbours have had twins. Hurray for them! I only realized this when I saw the little pairs of tights and dresses on the washing line – two pairs of everything, it's very cute. I'd like to think one of them is called Gemma, as I often hear "Gemma, don't do that" or "Gemma, you're such a good girl" but that could just be my imagination!

As I'm writing now, I can hear "Gemma" and her sister giggling through the terraced walls. Having them next door and hearing them laugh and cry is a little confronting. I'm forced to face the idea of motherhood and the regular inner conversation of whether I will ever be a mother.

Questioning decisions

When I was younger I said I didn't want children. I wanted to focus on my career. I do think a lot of this decision was based on losing Sean. Having him taken from my life was heartbreaking, but my pain can't compare to that of my mother. I just don't think I'm strong enough to experience that, and the thought of it terrifies me. I definitely have a fear of losing people close to me as a result of losing Sean.

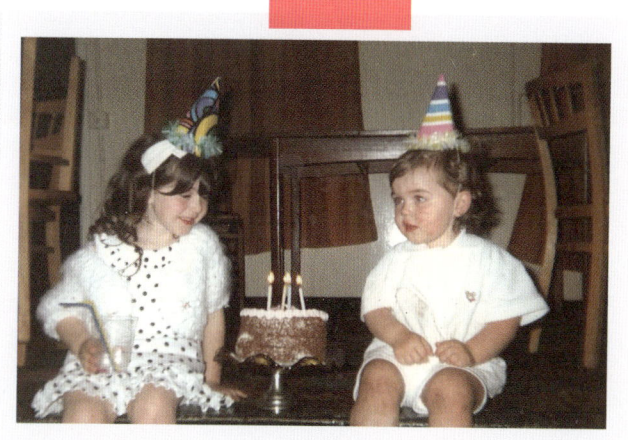

Of course, as I've got older I've questioned this decision. I watch the people around me build their own little families and it really does tug at my heart and play with my emotions, which range from smugness and relief to jealousy and bitterness. The family parties and the baby showers, they're all too much for me. I found myself at a christening a year ago with tears rolling down my face for the entire ceremony. I felt like I was crying for what I didn't have, but I still wasn't sure if that was what I wanted. I need to hurry up and make a decision; I'm running out of time! The questions from others as well as myself are endless, and the pressure can be overwhelming if I think about it too much. So, I try not to. Last year I was diagnosed with endometriosis, and this paired with my age could make it very difficult for me to conceive. It would seem the odds are against me ... although not impossible. What will be will be.

I do think I would make a good mother. The relationship I have with my own mother means everything to me and I would like to have that with my own child.

The idea of becoming a mother really does force me to look at myself, who I am and what I want from my life. When I'm having these conversations with myself, I like to look myself in the eye. However, I find it incredibly hard to look in the mirror for any real length of time. I can put my makeup on in the morning, point out my physical flaws and then go about my normal day. But to truly look at myself takes courage.

Every once in a while I will attempt my self-portrait. I find it easier to look at myself if it involves a task, such as painting. The process of drawing or painting myself allows me to self-reflect. Scrutinizing myself in such detail can be confronting, but it allows me to see myself – the good, the bad and the ugly.

SELF-PORTRAIT

A self-portrait is a perfect task when personal reflection and inner conversations are required. Creating a self-portrait can be a deeply personal and rewarding experience, whether you're a beginner or an experienced artist. I've found it a great exercise to help me look at my own reflection; it forces me to truly see myself – both the outside and the inside. It takes time and practice, but I try to embrace everything I see before me.

Please rest assured that this activity, like all the activities in this book, is for you to benefit from the process of creating; you don't necessarily have to love the final outcome. So I don't want you to worry about your skill set here. Self-portraits are one of the hardest things to create, as they require both technical skill and self-observation. Capturing a true likeness, understanding the proportions of the facial features, can take years of study and practice to get right. So, as beginners, let's not be too hard on ourselves. As you can see, my portrait is hardly a photograph!

I've been many different versions of myself throughout my 40 years. I've been lost, broken, withdrawn, hopeful, passionate, determined and quite often lonely. Today I look at myself and I see … a work in progress. I see the kindness in my eyes, I see the spark that was once lost, I see the excitement for the future, I see potential. I see the good and where I need to improve. I see what decisions I need to make.

My mum always says, if you don't know what to do, don't do anything and give yourself time. Motherhood is an uncertainty for me, so for now I will just keep looking within myself and one day (soon) I hope the answer will present itself.

Look within you … What emotions do you see? Calmness, sadness, hope? Look as much as you can. If you're anything like me, then capturing yourself on the page is another story altogether. But, like I keep saying, it's a process.

Creating each other's portraits is also an ideal group or even a date-night activity. Drawing or painting portraits allows for a more playful experience, and if your portrait skill set is on a par with mine then I'm certain it will be an activity full of giggles!

YOU WILL NEED

★ **A mirror** – or a photograph on your phone

★ **Paper, card, canvas** or **sketchbook**

★ **For drawing** – pens or pencils, eraser, sharpener

★ **For painting** – brushes and paints (acrylics are my go-to but you may want to use oil or watercolours), a palette for mixing your paints, a jar of water for cleaning brushes

HOW TO CREATE A SELF-PORTRAIT

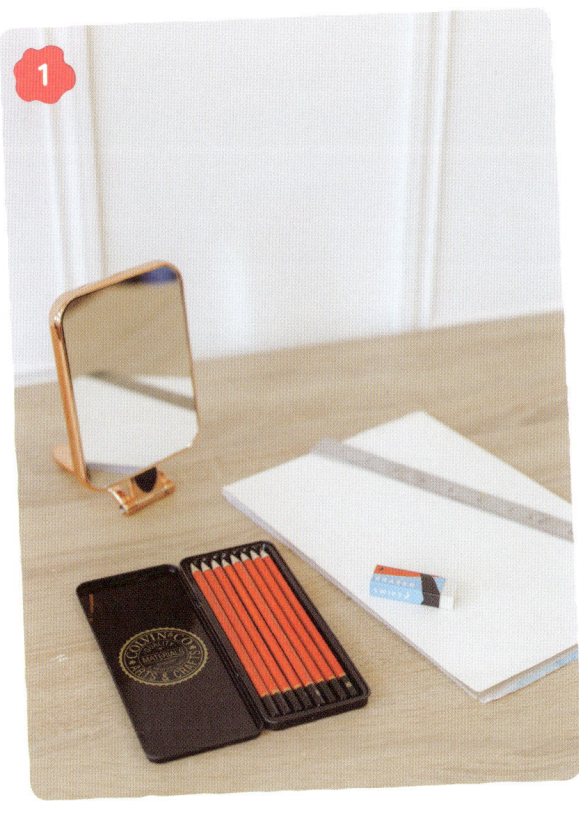

1. Look at yourself in the mirror. Sitting in a well-lit area is ideal for this activity, as you can see yourself clearly in all your natural beauty. Spend some time observing your face, looking at the shape, proportions and your unique features. Is your face oval, round or square? Look at the positioning and size of your eyes, nose, mouth and ears. Look at the structure of your bones and muscles, shadows and highlights.

2. Do a sketch. Whether I'm drawing or painting, I always find it useful to sketch out the portrait first in pencil. Starting with light lines to outline the basic shape of your head, divide the face into proportional sections using the guidelines below.

3. Draw a circle with a cross through it. The circle represents the top portion

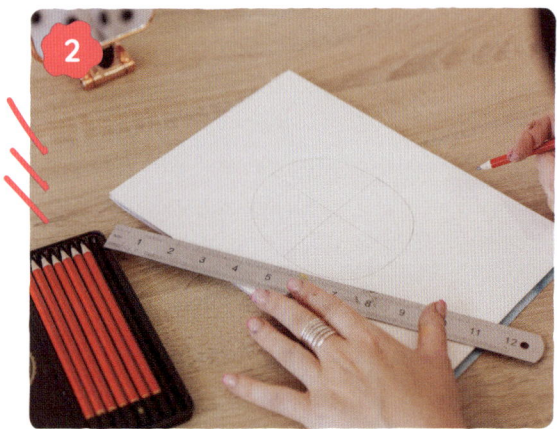

of the head, the cross will determine the locations of the facial features with the eyes on the line across the middle.

4. Draw a large square inside the circle. This square will eventually represent the edges of the face. The top line will become the bottom hairline. The bottom line will become the nose line.

5. Now draw the chin under the original circle. You can compare the distance from your eyes to the bottom of your nose, and from your nose to your chin using your pencil. Then use this measurement to mark the location of the bottom of the chin from the bottom line of the square. Then draw the edges of the chin from each side of the square so that they connect at your marked location.

6. Now that we have the basic structure of the face in place, we can start to draw in the details, starting with the eyes. We can use the height of the

Eyes: Pay close attention to the shape and details of the eyes. For a more detailed portrait or maybe even a close-up, include the iris, pupil and reflections.

Nose and mouth: Observe the unique shape and structure of your nose and lips. Notice the way light and shadow fall on these features.

Ears and hair: Include the shape of your ears and hair, paying attention to texture and volume.

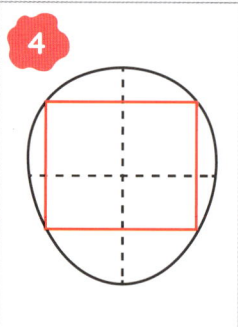
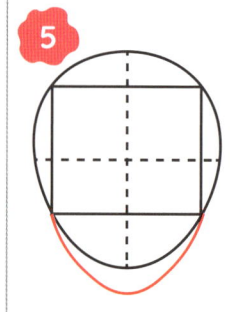
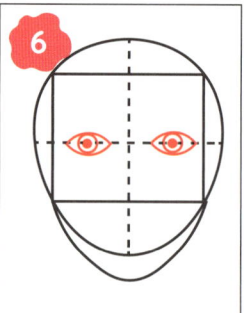
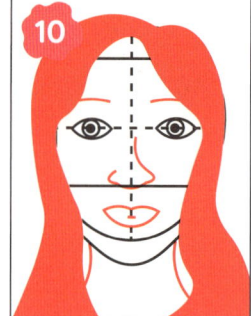

head to help us determine the location of the eyes on the face. The eyes are generally found on a line in the centre of the head. It also helps to consider the width of the eyes. The width of the head, from ear to ear, is generally the same length as five eyes.

7. Next, draw the nose. The bottom of the nose will sit on the bottom line of your square. The width of the nose varies from person to person but is generally as wide as the inside corners of the eyes.

8. Moving on to the mouth. You will find the mouth slightly higher than half-way between the bottom of the nose and the chin. Again, this varies from person to person.

9. The top of the ears will generally align with the brow line, while the bottom of the ears align with the nose line.

10. The face should now be starting to take shape and at least look like a person, if not exactly like you. The final part of the sketch will be the hair. If you have short hair then the hairline will be found on the top line of your square. If you have long hair, it's likely your hair will overlap this line.

You have a sketched self-portrait! You may wish to now spend some time adding in details using shading and texture to add depth and dimension.

If, like me, you're a colour lover, now would be a great time to introduce some colours. You can paint, use pastels, coloured pencils ... whatever takes your fancy.

⊕ I find producing a self-portrait a very personal experience; it forces you to look at who you are. The task itself is also a challenging one and doesn't come easily to many of us. I must admit I was a little embarrassed to show you all my self-portrait, as I feel it lacks in skill. But then I reminded myself to practise what I preach: it's the process, Gemma, and not the final outcome!

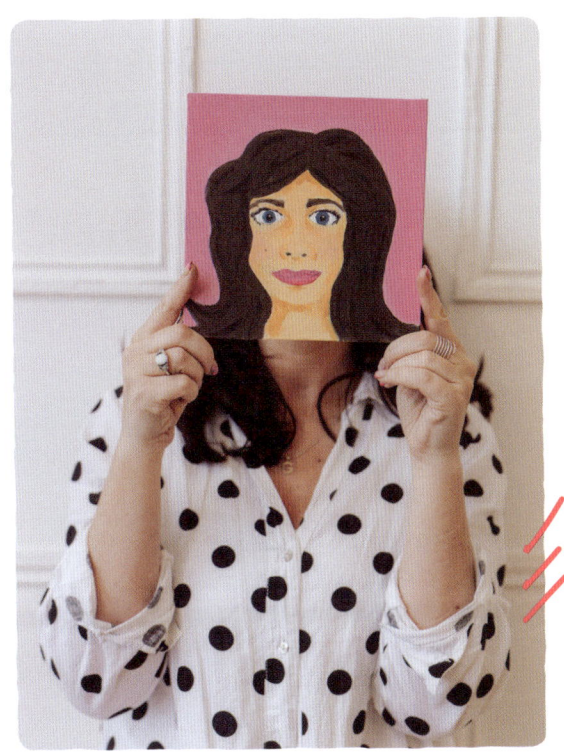

CELEBRATING SMALL WINS

As I'm sure you're all aware, postcards are generally used when we are away from the everyday. They capture special memories worth writing home about. They're like old-school social media; we use them to post our highlights, the best bits. So why not use them to celebrate our small wins in our day-to-day lives? I believe that recognizing and being grateful for the little things will make us more positive people and our self-esteem will increase.

I'm aware how old it makes me sound when I say that when I was younger we didn't have camera phones to take and send photographs. There was no uploading our whereabouts and holiday snaps to social media. We had to use actual cameras and get the photographs developed when we returned home – I know, what a faff!

But, of course, there was always the good old-fashioned postcard to let the folks back home know how much of a great time we were having – although we probably could have just told them ourselves, as more often than not we would arrive home before the postcard did!

Postcards tell of our holiday highlights – the fancy restaurants, the beachside hotel, the beautiful weather. We don't tend to write home about all the things that have gone wrong! In a way, postcards are just like Instagram, where we only post the things we are most proud of – the beautifully styled home, the delicious home-cooked meal, the expensive outfit and the lavish holiday. We don't show the mess on the other side of the camera, all the other home-cooked meals that we've burnt, or the fact that we've spent most of the day in our tracksuit bottoms and not that expensive outfit.

Yes, we certainly do have our highlights, but if we're honest, the majority of our days are not Instagram or postcard worthy.

Overcoming dark days

Today I am proud that I have overcome some very dark days, glad that I didn't give in and grateful for the strength and passion I have. Today is postcard worthy, it's certainly a highlight of my story … Today I am writing a book!

My goodness, it's been a journey to get to this day, a journey filled with mostly average and rather boring days, more sad days than good, as well as a lot of loneliness and confusion. It's on these mundane and often gloomy days that I feel it's important to celebrate the small wins, the tiny steps that we make on our path to recovery.

When my depression was at its worst, doing anything noteworthy was absolutely out of the question. Simply washing my hair was something to be celebrated. Making sure I ate a proper meal and getting through the day were my priority, and a lot of the time even those fell to my mum, as all I was capable of was breathing. On the lighter days, I walked the dog and did the dishes, and as the number of lighter days increased, I could talk on the phone and eventually made a button necklace.

These insignificant tasks kept me going and are to be celebrated.

Everyday moments

Life is a little overwhelming for me at the moment, in a good way. I'm doing my best to run my own business, live my dream, tell my story and share my passions all whilst keeping my head above water, paying the bills, cleaning the house, being a good friend, girlfriend and daughter, and staying fit and healthy both physically and mentally. I'm not complaining, but it can sometimes be hard, especially as an independent woman. I'm doing my best, and most days I nail it. However, I can suffer from burnout and there are days when I have to stay in bed, switch off and do NOTHING!

On these days, just getting out of bed is worth celebrating. So, I want to honour these crucial small wins, the small yet huge steps we make in our everyday lives. Today I made … a postcard!

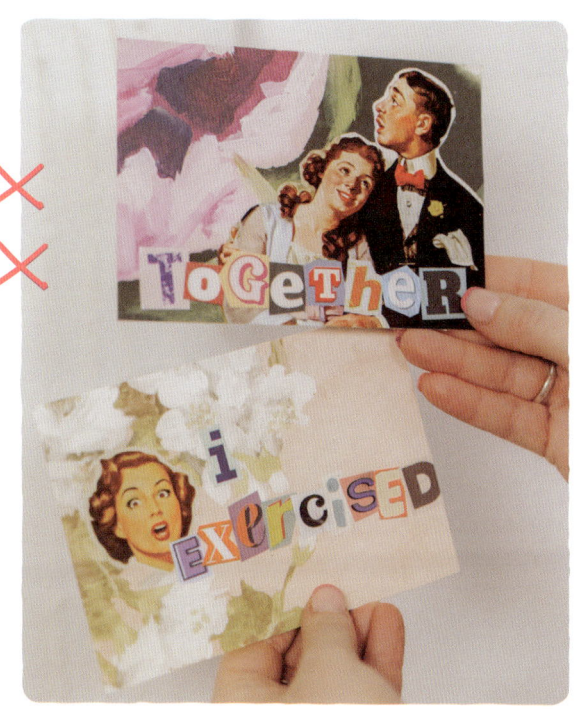

COLLAGE POSTCARD

This task allows you to be in the moment while acknowledging and celebrating a particular highlight. By thinking about the importance of your actions, however small they may seem, you'll find that you're more present as you go about your day.

Making a postcard is relatively quick and won't take up too much of your energy – the perfect task for the days when you're lacking in motivation. Doing this every so often will mean one small step will soon grow into a larger story that tells a tale. The idea of small individual tasks making up a bigger picture is why I feel collage is the perfect medium for these postcards; there is a connection between the medium and action. Collage is an art technique that involves creating an image or composition using various materials and elements, such as photographs, magazine clippings, paper, fabric and found objects. The word "collage" derives from the French word *coller*, which means "to glue".

I often cut letters out of magazines as I read them and keep them ready to go at such moments as this. I love a charity shop haul and often find lots of old unwanted books with some fabulous photos. The older the book, the more aged the paper looks, and I love that – the creamy beige colour and musty dusty pages tear beautifully!

YOU WILL NEED

★ **Blank postcard** or cardboard cut to size – the standard size for a postcard is 10cm x 15cm/4in x 6in

★ **Scrap papers, magazines, newspapers**

★ **Glue** – PVA or Pritt stick is ideal

★ **Scissors** or craft knife

HOW TO MAKE A POSTCARD

1. Think of what you would like to celebrate: getting out of bed, paying the gas bill, driving to the shop. I'm celebrating the fact that I did a little exercise – a win for me, as it happens very rarely!

2. Cut, tear, rip out images from your magazines and newspapers that mean something to you and simply compile them together. I've managed to find a lady looking shocked, which is the ideal expression considering how infrequently I exercise.

3. Design your postcard by arranging your cut-outs on the postcard, starting with the background and placing your message or images over the top. I cover the entire surface of the postcard for a more effective look. I find it helps to place all the images down first before sticking, so that I can work out the best composition.

4. Once you're happy with your arrangement, apply your glue evenly to the back of your cut-outs and stick down firmly.

5. Pop your postcard somewhere you can see it or maybe send it to someone or even yourself as

a reminder of how well you're doing. Keep going. You're doing great!

⊕ This is a super-easy, quick craft that gets your hands moving, your creativity flowing and forces you to think a little more positively about yourself. If all you did today was make this postcard, GO YOU!

Creating collage artwork is a fun and versatile artistic process that allows for endless experimentation and creativity. Don't be afraid to try new techniques, mix different materials and let your imagination run wild as you explore the possibilities of collage-making. Working on a larger scale is lots of fun, but that's for another day. Today we celebrate the little things.

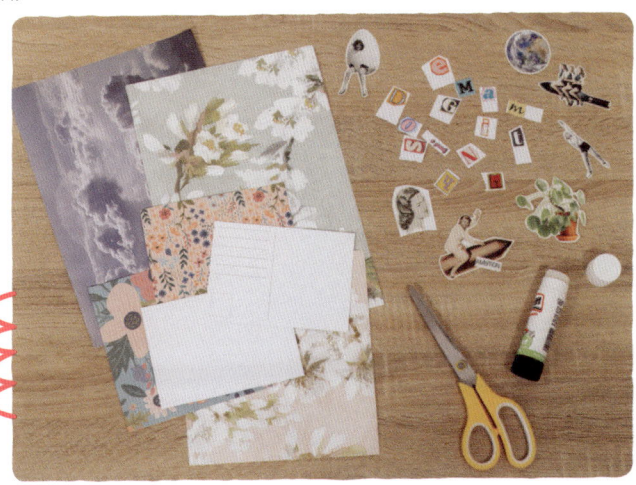

EXPRESSIVE PAINTING

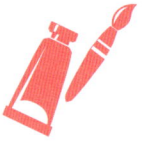

Painting is definitely my favourite medium when it comes to being creative. It's messy, transformative, colourful and playful. For me, it's the perfect medium for expressing emotions as it allows you to be playful and experimental with colours, mark-making, tools and techniques.

Expressive painting is abstract in style, spontaneous and deeply personal to the creator. It allows the artist to convey emotions, feelings and personal experiences through bold brushstrokes, vibrant colours and dynamic compositions. An expressive painting captures the energy and essence of the artist's mood during its creation.

What I love about expressive painting is that anyone can do it. You don't need to be particularly talented to create something special and meaningful.

I'm no Picasso, but that doesn't stop me from expressing myself and making my mark through the medium of paint – and it shouldn't stop you either!

Making my mark

Expressive painting is freeing – there are no rules! I remember the first time

I experienced this freedom to paint. It was one summer's day when Sean and I were at my grandparents' house. My grandad had the most awesome garden shed, which he built himself using scrap wood, an old window and a front door. He had all sorts in the shed, he didn't like to throw anything away. Anyway, on this lovely summer's day my grandad gave me some tester pots of paint he had been storing in his shed, an array of colours from previous decorating projects. He said to do anything I wanted with them …

I spent this beautiful day painting flowers all over the garden, on pretty much every surface I could find. The walls, fence, doors … I really went for it. Well, he did say I could do anything! It was one of the happiest days of my childhood, painting pink and purple flowers in my childlike style while the sun shone down on me. I look back and think this was the first day I was able to truly make my mark with paint. Of course, I loved what I had created. From where I was standing, I had brought happiness to their garden, and my grandparents clearly agreed, as they never painted over it.

Today I regularly paint; it's my way to let off steam. If I've had a tough day at work, I paint. If I'm feeling stressed and overwhelmed with life, I paint. If I'm sad, anxious, stressed, excited, relieved … I paint! I just love to paint.

Most of the time when I start to paint, I'm thinking to myself, *This won't work, you're too stressed*. But without fail, I start to relax and my busy mind calms. My stresses and worries of the day fade and my thoughts turn to the composition on the canvas, the colours that I'm using and brushstrokes I'm creating.

Saved by paint

I was rescued by paint a few Decembers ago, when I was feeling rather down. I'd recently come out of a long-term relationship. I was living in a new home in a different part of the city. I had distanced myself from the few friends I had. Work was slow and I had very little money, and as a result of this I felt isolated and alone – and of course it always feels worse at Christmas.

It's just me and my mum at Christmas now. Please don't get me wrong, I adore my mum and truly appreciate how lucky I am to get to spend Christmas with her. But binge-watching *Bridgerton* on Christmas Day with your mum is pretty awkward, as handsome as the duke is!

I've always dreamed of being a part of a big family at Christmas – everyone sitting around the table tucking into Christmas dinner, laughing, pulling crackers and telling jokes.

That year, I had no plans for New Year's Eve. It felt like everyone around me was happy; they all had their families, their partners or their parties to go to. My plan was to go to bed early and avoid the entire thing. I didn't want to hear the clock strike 12, feel the twang of disappointment that there was no one there to kiss and the fear and uncertainty of what the new year would bring for me.

But in a moment of courage, I changed my mind. Knowing what I know about painting and the beneficial impact it can have on my mood encouraged my change of heart. Instead of going to bed, I decided to paint. I got a few canvases out, put on my favourite playlist and painted the new year in. Admittedly it started off forced and reluctant, but I soon got into it. I used all my favourite paints and brushes and turned the evening around.

I saw in the new year with three beautiful expressive canvases. Now hanging on my wall at home, those canvases represent a huge transformation – the night I left behind my lonely days and welcomed a fresh start and positive future.

INNER MASTERPIECE

Expressive painting is so much fun and can be really freeing. If you're feeling a little low, deflated or stressed, this activity is for you. Be open-minded and push past the overthinking. You will be glad you did.

For some people, expressive painting takes time to get into. I've found through delivering painting workshops that children respond best to the lack of structure and freedom to play; adults, however, are in need of direction, a goal or a reference for comparison, and can even be terrified by the very idea of this!

So, to start with, you need to clear your mind of any sort of outcome for your painting. Giving yourself an end goal will limit your playful intuitive nature. Expressive painting allows you to play with mark-making, which is why I like to introduce as many tools to paint with as possible. I love using found or scrap materials; my favourites are torn papers, bubble wrap and tooth brushes. Experiment and explore what marks can be created with whatever materials you have to hand.

YOU WILL NEED

★ **A surface** to paint on – canvas, paper, cardboard

★ **Easel** – not necessary, but it can be helpful

★ **Paint** – ANY! This activity is all about mark-making, so anything will do. Acrylics are ideal but a few tester pots will also work well.

★ **Paint brushes** – a range of sizes would be perfect

Warning! This exercise can be messy, so protect yourself and your surroundings by putting covers down and wearing appropriate clothing. You want to be able to express yourself without worrying about your favourite top getting paint on it.

★ **Sponges**

★ **Scrap materials** – cardboard, paper and bubble wrap are all great for printing

★ **Palette knives**

★ **Palette** – you can buy pads of palette paper, which I use a lot, but a piece of card, an old plate or a food container lid works just as well

★ **Spray bottle**

★ **Jar of water** – for cleaning brushes

★ **A hairdryer** – handy for drying off your canvas in between layers. It speeds up the process.

HOW TO CREATE AN INNER MASTERPIECE

1. Gather all your materials. It's a good idea to have everything to hand rather than running around the house halfway through painting to find something ... It kinda ruins the vibe.

2. Choose your colour palette. How are you feeling? What colours would you like to use to reflect this? Now is a great time to refer back to the colour psychology section at the beginning of the book (see pages 14–15).

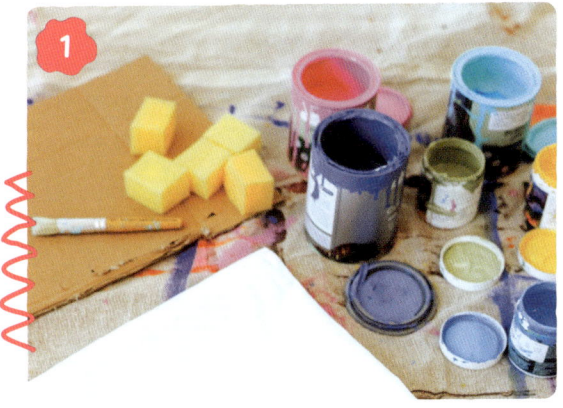

3. Get some paint on the canvas. A blank canvas can be daunting, so just start, don't overthink it. Start by adding brushstrokes to your canvas with various brushes and colours. Be playful and use big, bold strokes.

4. Dry with the hairdryer.

5. Start building texture and depth using your scrap materials. Paint the edge of a piece of cardboard, some bubble wrap, or some scrunched-up paper and print with them. Build up your layers, drying in between.

6. Explore different paint techniques such as dripping the paint onto the canvas and splatting. Using

watered-down paint in a spray bottle achieves some great effects and it's lots of fun to do!

TIP: While you're painting, think about the composition and the balance of your painting - how does it work visually? This is all personal preference; some love symmetry while others like to build up one area of the canvas, but it's worth thinking about as you add each layer.

7. Try using your palette knife to apply paint thickly to the canvas, or try scratching the paint with the edge of the knife.

8. Sponges are great for blending colours together and creating an ombré effect.

9. Keep building on your layers, adding more depth and colour to your composition with each mark that you make. Embrace your "mistakes". Remember, there are no mistakes when it comes to this style of painting.

10. Once you feel like your canvas is complete, then stop. Take a minute to appreciate what you have created. Reflect on the marks that you have made and the intention behind each of them.

⊕ Hopefully at the end of this process you will have created something beautifully unique to you and allowed your tired, over-stimulated mind some recovery time. Your mood will have lifted and you will be full of inspiration for your next painting experience.

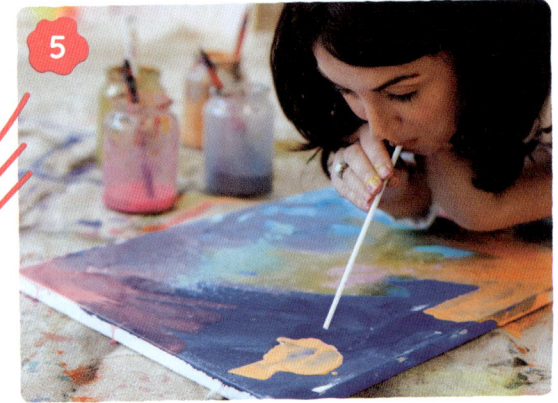

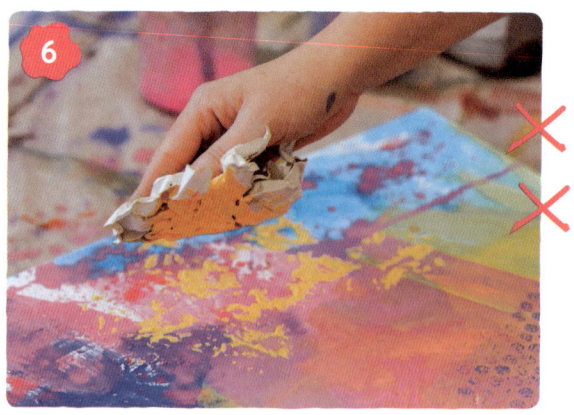

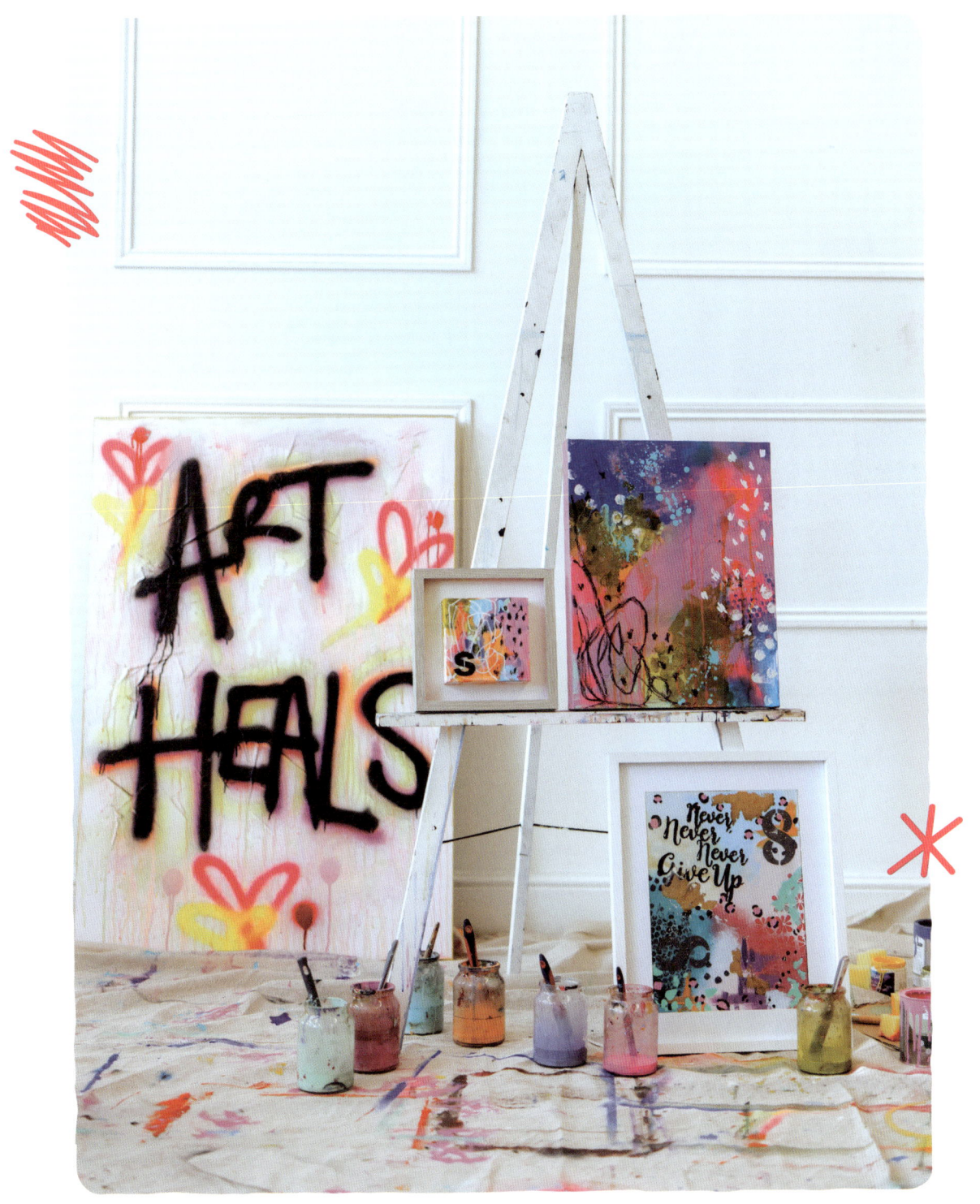

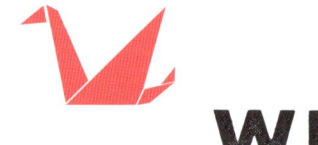 # FOCUS WITH FOLDING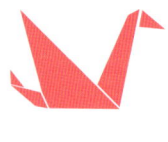

Origami is the traditional Japanese art of paper folding, where *ori* means "folding" and *kami* means "paper". It involves transforming a flat sheet of paper into a finished sculpture through folding and sculpting techniques. It's great for our mental health, as it reduces stress, promotes concentration and even improves cognitive function.

The most important person to me is my mum! Her name is Julie, but we all call her Lee. Lee is the most kind-hearted, amazing person you will ever meet, and I am so fortunate to have her in my life. There is nothing I wouldn't do for her and vice versa, although if she asks me to wallpaper her bathroom one more time I will have to have words!

My mum married my dad in 1981 in a blue wedding dress and with a tight perm. Three years later, on 12 May 1984, I was born and three years after that, on 24 April 1987, Sean was born. My parents divorced in 1995, which is not my story to tell, so I will leave that there. Of course, divorce is extremely hard, and my mum struggled to bring Sean and me up on a shoestring budget. None of this could have been easy for her, but what she faced next was so much worse. The

following year Sean died. I can't imagine the pain she must have felt.

Mum and me

My mum and I have been through so much together and as a result we have the utmost respect and love for each other. We speak to each other every day and we only have to utter one word over the phone for the other to know exactly how we are feeling. Lee has been through so much heartache and I can't believe how she's got through it and is still the beautiful person that she is.

I firmly believe that if you don't like my mum then there is something wrong with you.

Lee comes along to many of my workshops and classes to help and spend time with me. I work a lot, so it's often her chance for us to be together. People warm to her instantly. She puts everyone at ease, makes them feel good about themselves, is super friendly and has a brilliant sense of humour. She's a little mood-booster in stonewashed denim and sparkly Sketchers.

After losing Sean, I've become her everything. She's my biggest cheerleader and ALWAYS has my back. She's like a lioness protecting her cub. If you dare to upset me … Well, don't say I didn't warn you. If someone has the nerve to dislike me or disagree with me, then according to her they must be jealous!

My relationship with my mother certainly makes up for the lack of other relationships in my life. However, I am aware how much pressure this puts on our bond. Heaven forbid anything happens to either of us, because the other just couldn't cope. A little more security in my life would benefit us both, as my mum wouldn't worry about me as much.

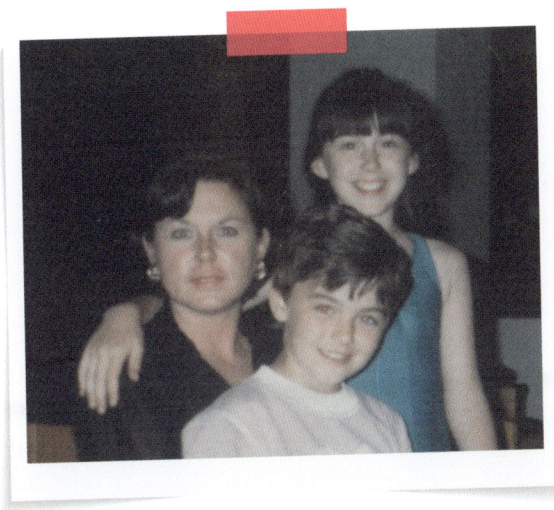

Special gifts

When it comes to showing my mum how much I love her, nothing I can buy will say enough. My time and my thoughts are the only things that portray this. That's why I believe gifting something handmade brings so much more joy and conveys so much more than something shop-bought.

We all have busy lives, so taking the time to hand-make something for a loved one is a precious gift in my book … and this is my book!

My mum has kept almost everything I've ever made for her. She still has the giant paper snowflake I made for her in primary school and she proudly puts it on the Christmas tree every year – although as I've got older, it has made its way to the back of the tree … She's very particular with her Christmas tree!

I hope I'm not giving away my mum's secrets here, but she has been known to wrap up empty boxes to put under the Christmas tree so the tree looks perfect even when all the presents have been unwrapped. She matches the wrapping paper to her baubles and everything is colour-coordinated. It does look beautiful. As you can probably tell, gift wrapping is very important in our house, and when it comes to gift wrapping, there is nothing better than a handmade gift box. It's the kind of thing you can use time and time again.

ORIGAMI GIFT BOX

Here we're making a handmade gift box with origami, which is such a lovely way to present your gift and shows just how much thought you have put into it.

While paper-folding traditions have existed in many cultures, origami as it is known today is most closely associated with Japan. The practice dates to the 17th century but is still super popular today. Japanese origami was originally used to decorate temples and shrines, but you can make so many amazing things – from animals to flowers and even people! Because it requires minimal materials, it's a perfect craft for anyone and everyone.

This project is a great way to use up old papers such as magazines and wallpaper, but you can also use photocopied photographs and dated newspapers for that sentimental touch.

There are many crafts in this book that would make wonderful gifts to put in the box, such as the button jewellery on pages 100–2 or the clay keepsakes on pages 132–4.

YOU WILL NEED

★ **2 x square pieces of paper** – mine measure 30cm x 30cm/12in x 12in, but you can use a larger or small piece depending on what size box you're going for. One piece of paper will be for the base of the box and the other for the lid of the box. Sugar paper, gift wrap and standard copy paper are all great. Tissue paper is too thin and cardboard is too thick.

★ Ruler

★ Pencil

★ **Craft knife** or **scissors**

HOW TO MAKE AN ORIGAMI GIFT BOX

1. Using your ruler, draw an X from corner to corner on the BACK of your paper. These are the fold lines. Take your time and make sure to get them exactly centred. If they're not, the folds you make will be uneven and your box will be a bit wonky.

2. Position the paper into a diamond shape in front of you, and then fold each corner into the centre of the X. Again, make sure they meet perfectly for your box to turn out symmetrical.

3. Unfold the corners and open out the paper. Then take each corner and fold up past the centre to your new fold line on the opposite side. Repeat for each corner.

4. Open up the paper again. You will see lots of fold lines.

5. Take one corner again and fold it into the original centre point. This time you will fold the tip of triangle back on itself to meet the middle of your folded line.

6. Repeat for every corner.

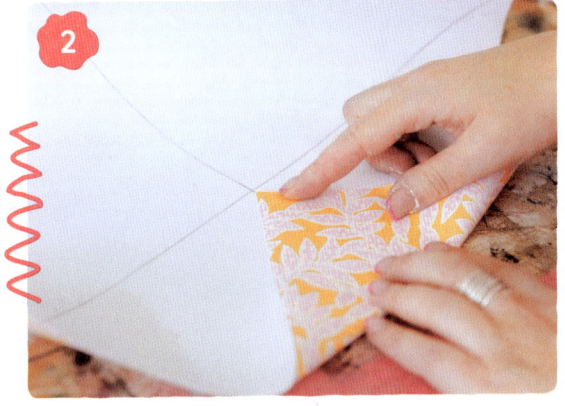

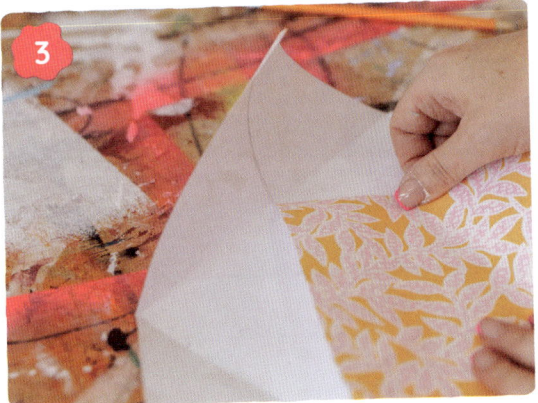

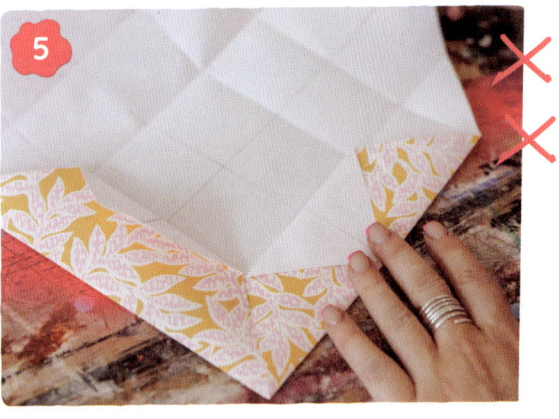

7. Unfold the top and bottom, leaving the two sides folded in.

8. Lift the two folded sides upwards to form the first two sides of your box.

9. Keeping those sides upright, fold over the top and bottom to create the third and fourth sides of your box. This can be a little tricky. It's an "in and over" motion. Allow the paper to fold back into the folded lines you have created.

10. Press all your folds into place to secure your box.

That's the top of the box done!

TIP: You can glue down the folds if you feel your box needs it. This will depend on what you will be storing inside your box. Heavier items may require glue, as they will put pressure on the folds.

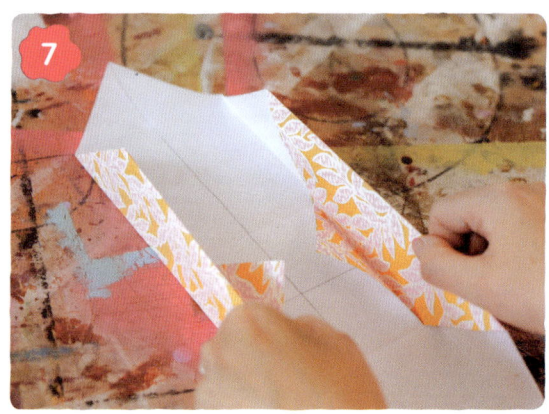

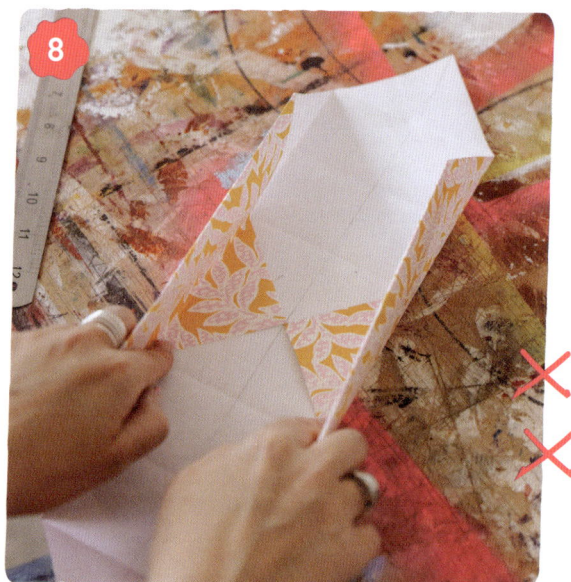

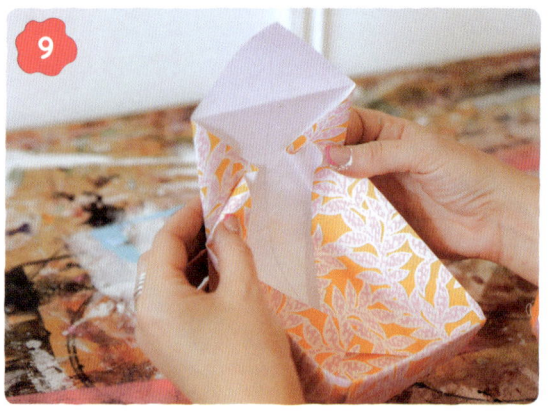

11. Repeat all the steps again, with a slightly smaller piece of paper – cut off 3mm/⅛in off the height and width of your original measurements. This will make the base of your box. When finished, the top and base will fit snugly together into a beautiful, sturdy gift box.

Fancy making a bow to match? There's a template on page 177 …

12. Using the template, cut out the pieces for your bow in your decorative paper.

13. Add glue to the end of the larger piece (A). Fold both ends inwards and secure into the middle.

14. Take your folded piece (A) and attach to piece (B) by gluing in the middle.

15. Wrap piece (C) to middle and glue in place to form your perfect little bow.

16. Stick your bow to your gorgeous handmade box.

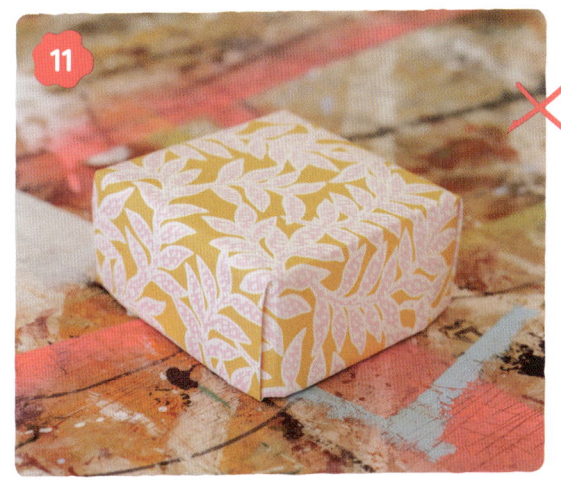

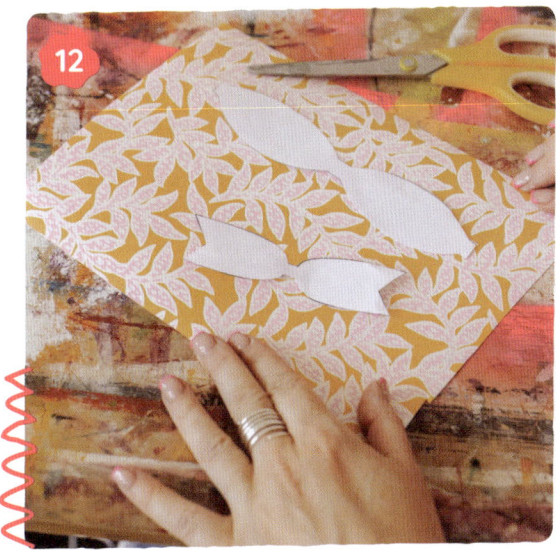

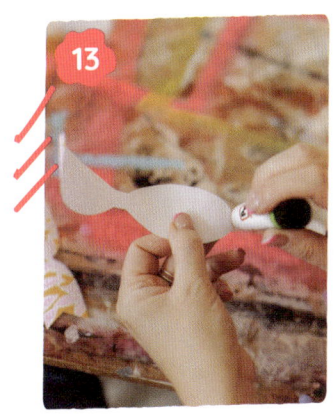

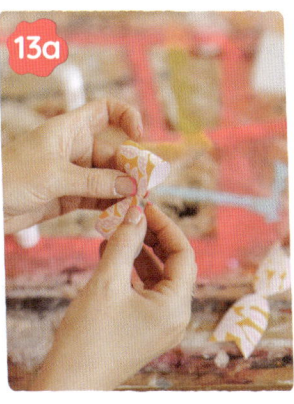

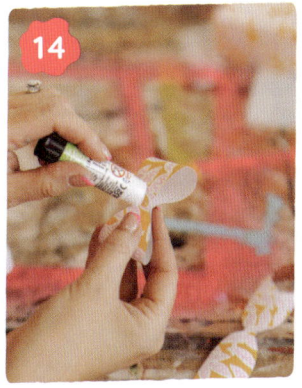

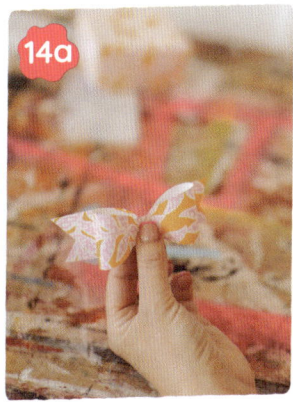

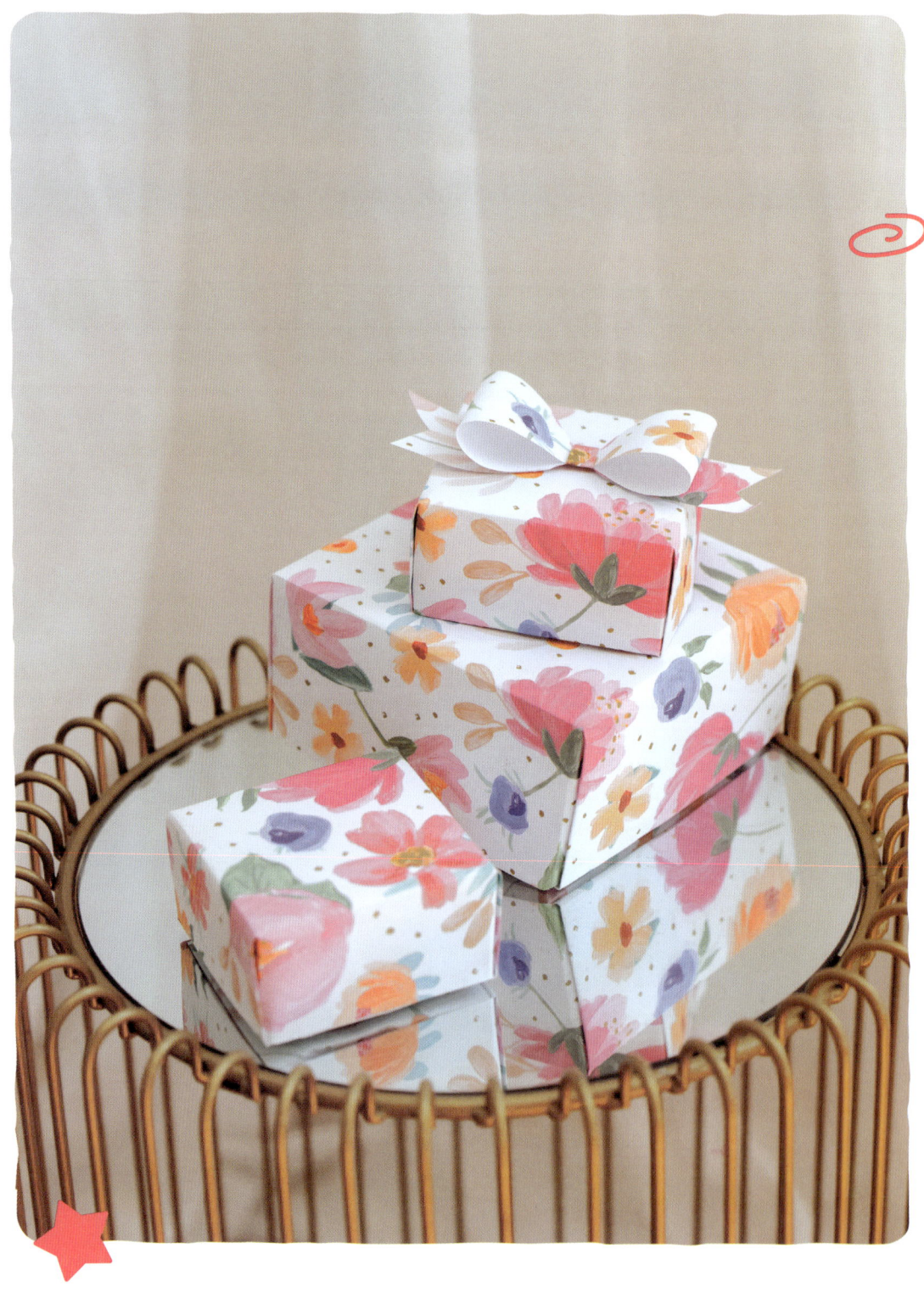

VISUAL AFFIRMATIONS

Words of affirmation can do wonders for us. Research has shown that daily positive self-affirmations – short positive statements – can reduce self-doubt and negative thoughts and boost our self-esteem. Not only can they have a powerful impact on our mental health and our confidence, they can also attract more positivity into our lives!

We've all seen the TV shows where the experts encourage us to look at ourselves in the mirror and tell ourselves how utterly wonderful we are. Now, is it just me or does the thought of this make you want to cringe?! But according to the experts we should all be talking to ourselves much more positively than we currently do.

Now, I know you may often feel quite the opposite of wonderful, beautiful, strong and loved. I must admit I find it easier to tell myself how rubbish I am. I struggle with my confidence and definitely suffer from imposter syndrome. I'm in a constant battle with myself to overcome the negative commentary.

I'm always the first to put myself down. I do it all the time and in front of other people too. It's my way of letting them know I'm aware of my failings, so they don't need to point them out. I've always been a sensitive soul. I take criticism personally and bat away the compliments, finding it much easier to believe the negative comments over the positive.

We believe what we hear

A few years back I noticed my confidence had plummeted. I found myself in a pretty toxic relationship in which I was constantly being put down. Negative comments were cast daily and were becoming increasingly more and more damaging. I didn't seem to notice at the time, but now that I'm away from this relationship I realize just how it affected my self-esteem. Nothing I did was good enough – the way I dressed, the job I chose, my cooking, my financial decisions. He would say I didn't have enough friends because I wasn't a nice person, that my family were overbearing and I needed to break free from them. I was a liar, I was stupid … I couldn't even paint my nails without a comment being made on my poor choice of colour; there was only one colour that was deemed acceptable! After we broke up, I went through a phase of painting my nails in crazy colours and patterns in rebellion.

It really infuriates me to look back now and think how I was manipulated to believe that I wasn't good enough. But if you hear something often enough, then you start to believe it. Of course that works for both positive and negative comments, which is why our positive daily affirmations are so important.

It's only been in the last few years that I've really started to notice that my internal monologue is having a damaging impact, that my overly sensitive nature is feeding my lack of self-confidence, leading to often severe anxiety. This really doesn't work when you have a job to do, a story to tell and passion to share with the world. I'm sure you've heard the saying, "Feel the fear and do it anyway" – well, that has been the story of my life for the last couple of years. I've been waking up each day with my stomach in knots!

Turning things around

I've recently made a conscious decision to surround myself with positivity, positive people and positive words. I've started to embrace self-affirmations and I really encourage you to do the same.

I'm drawing a line under my detrimental negative thoughts.

THE LINE

It's not going to be easy, so I'll need constant little reminders – and what better way to do this than with a handmade banner! So, let's go on this journey together and start talking to ourselves more positively. Even if we don't believe it wholeheartedly at first, let's do it anyway.

APPLIQUÉ BANNERS

Decorative banners are often used for celebrations, special events and occasions, but I believe our mental health is something to be celebrated. So we are going to create a positive-affirmation banner while taking part in a mindfulness activity. Sounds like a win-win to me.

First of all, what is appliqué, I hear you ask? Appliqué is a decorative technique in which pieces of fabric are sewn onto a larger fabric or garment to create a design or pattern. The term "appliqué" comes from the French word *appliquer*, which means "to apply" or "to put on". Appliqué can be used to embellish clothing, quilts, home décor items and more, such as affirmation banners!

There are many ways to create banners – painting, drawing and sewing, to name a few. On this occasion we will sew. Sewing is a great mindfulness activity that allows us to slow down.

Engaging in the repetitive motions of stitching can be meditative and calming, helping to reduce stress and anxiety.

Sewing projects can take a little longer to complete than painting or drawing. So the sense of accomplishment, whether it's a simple repair or a more intricate creation, can boost feelings of satisfaction and achievement. Seeing physical results of your efforts can increase self-esteem, and that's what this activity is all about. Confidently celebrating YOU.

YOU WILL NEED

★ **Fabric** – you will need a base fabric which the banner will be made out of, and a contrasting fabric(s) for your affirmation to allow it to stand out; we want to make a statement here, not blend into the background. Cottons, canvas, felt and polyester are good choices for this type of project. This might be a good opportunity to refer back to our colour theory. How do we want this banner to make us feel and what colour do we associate with these feelings? I love polka dots, leopard print and PINK, so let's include them all!

- ★ **Fusible webbing/interfacing** – a thin adhesive material that bonds fabric layers together when heated with an iron

- ★ **Scissors** – sharp fabric scissors

- ★ **Iron and ironing board**

- ★ **Needle and thread** – if you're hand-stitching your appliqué pieces

- ★ **String**, **wire** or **magnetic hanger**

If you want to go all out and get fancy pants, you can use trimming and finishing tools such as a rotary cutter, cutting mat, ruler and fabric marker for precise cutting and trimming of the appliqué pieces. If you have the banner bug, then why not?

HOW TO MAKE AN APPLIQUÉ BANNER

1. To start, create a design: plan out your banner first. How do you want your banner to make you feel? What saying makes you feel good and motivates you? In Liverpool we like to use "boss" when something is good. So I'm going to appliqué "you're boss" – which translates to "you're fab" – onto my banner. Draw this out on paper first.

2. Cut your background fabric to shape and size.

3. You may want to hem or stitch around the edges to create a neat finish.

4. Fold over the top and stitch. A basic running stitch approximately 2cm/1in in is ideal. This will allow you to add string or wire to your banner for hanging.

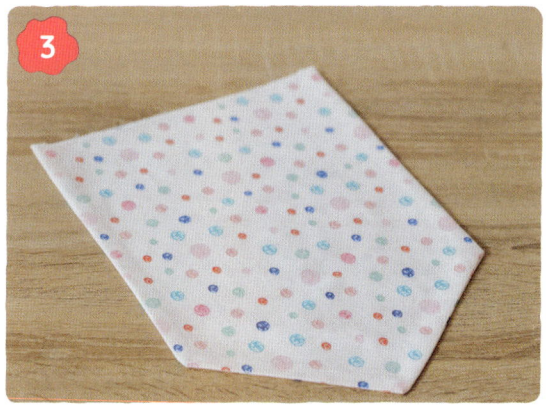

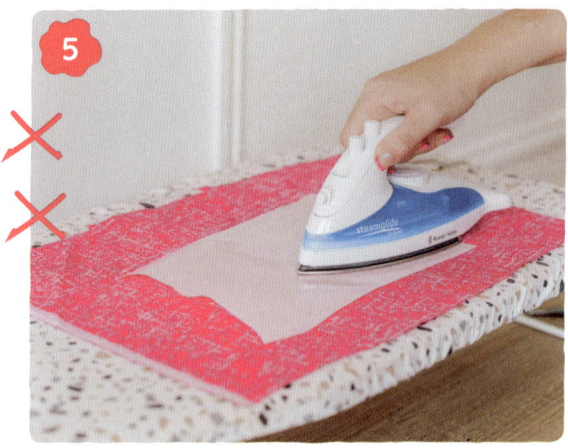

5. Take the fabric you will be using for your affirmation letters and iron the interfacing onto the back of this fabric. This will make your fabric feel stiff and almost paper-like and will help to hold our affirmation letters in place before stitching.

6. Draw the letters onto the back of the interfacing. Remember these will be reversed when ironed onto the banner, so you will have to draw the letters the wrong way round. If it's easier, you can cut out the letters from your paper design and use them as a template for your fabric letters.

7. Cut out all the fabric letters and remove the interface backing. This will leave a dry glue on the back of your fabric. This can be fiddly, especially for the nail biters, so be patient.

8. Lay out your cut-out fabric letters onto the background fabric, then iron in place. The heat from the iron will activate the glue and bond the two fabrics together. Your design should now be securely stuck down.

9. With the fabrics secure, you can now stitch around the edges of the letters using a simple ladder stitch. You can use a sewing machine for this, but I prefer the slower pace of hand-stitching. I will use different colour threads on each of the letters.

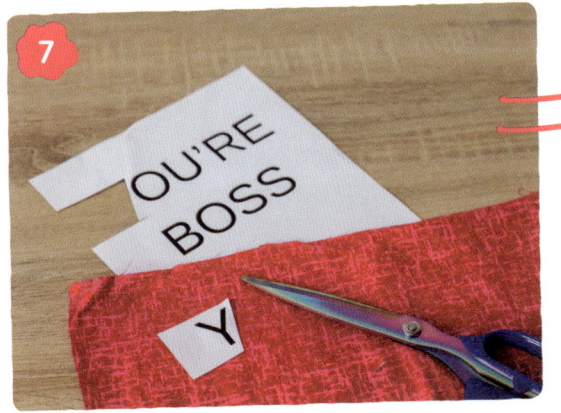

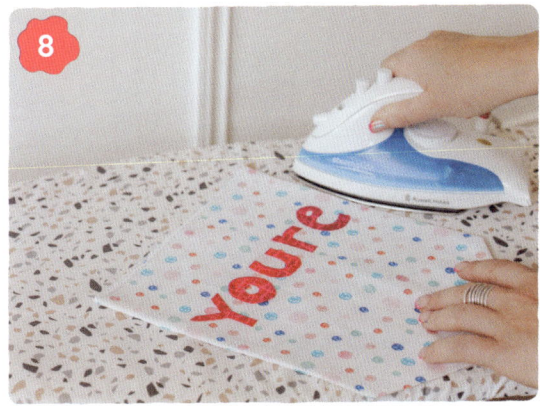

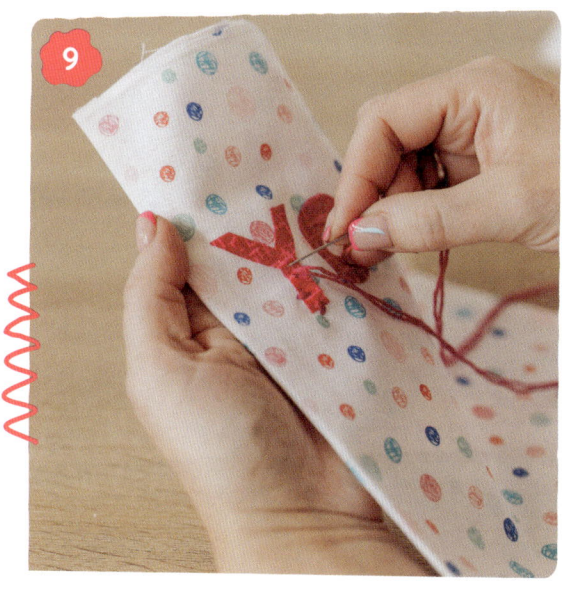

10. You can now hang or mount your banner. Thread a piece of string or wire through the top fold and use this to hang, or use a magnetic hanger as I've done here. Alternately these banners look great inside frames or embroidery hoops.

Your banner is technically complete although i've decided to go a step further and add a strip of pompoms to the bottom with a hot glue gun … a bit of shimmy, lace or feathers would also look fabulous.

11. Hang with pride, put it somewhere you will see it regularly, and every time you see it say the words out loud as a reminder of how fantastic you really are!

GEMMA, YOU'RE BOSS!

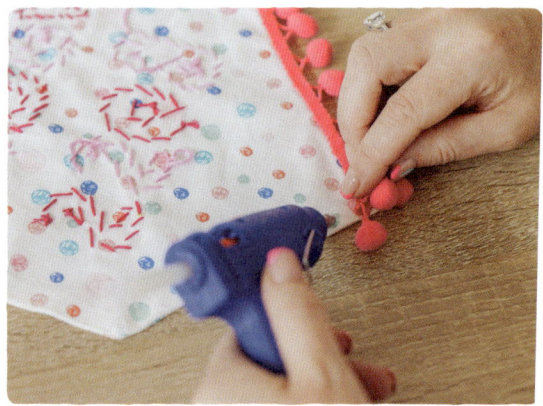

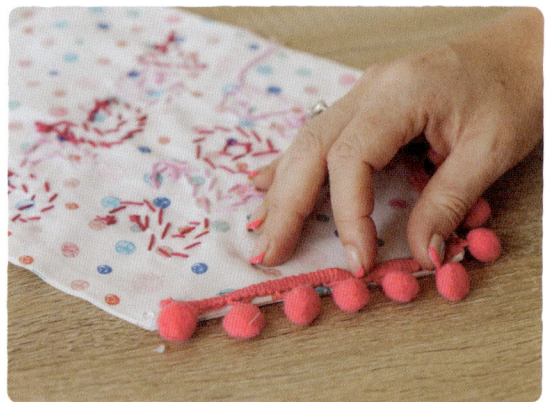

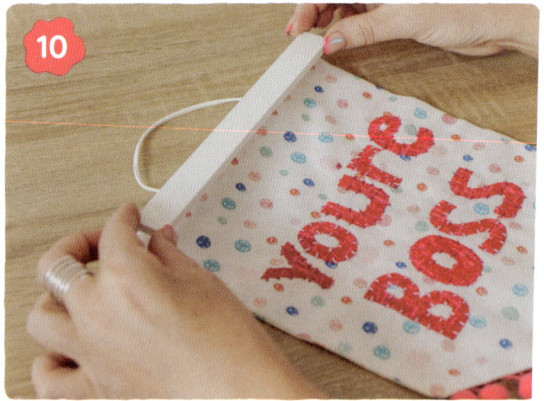

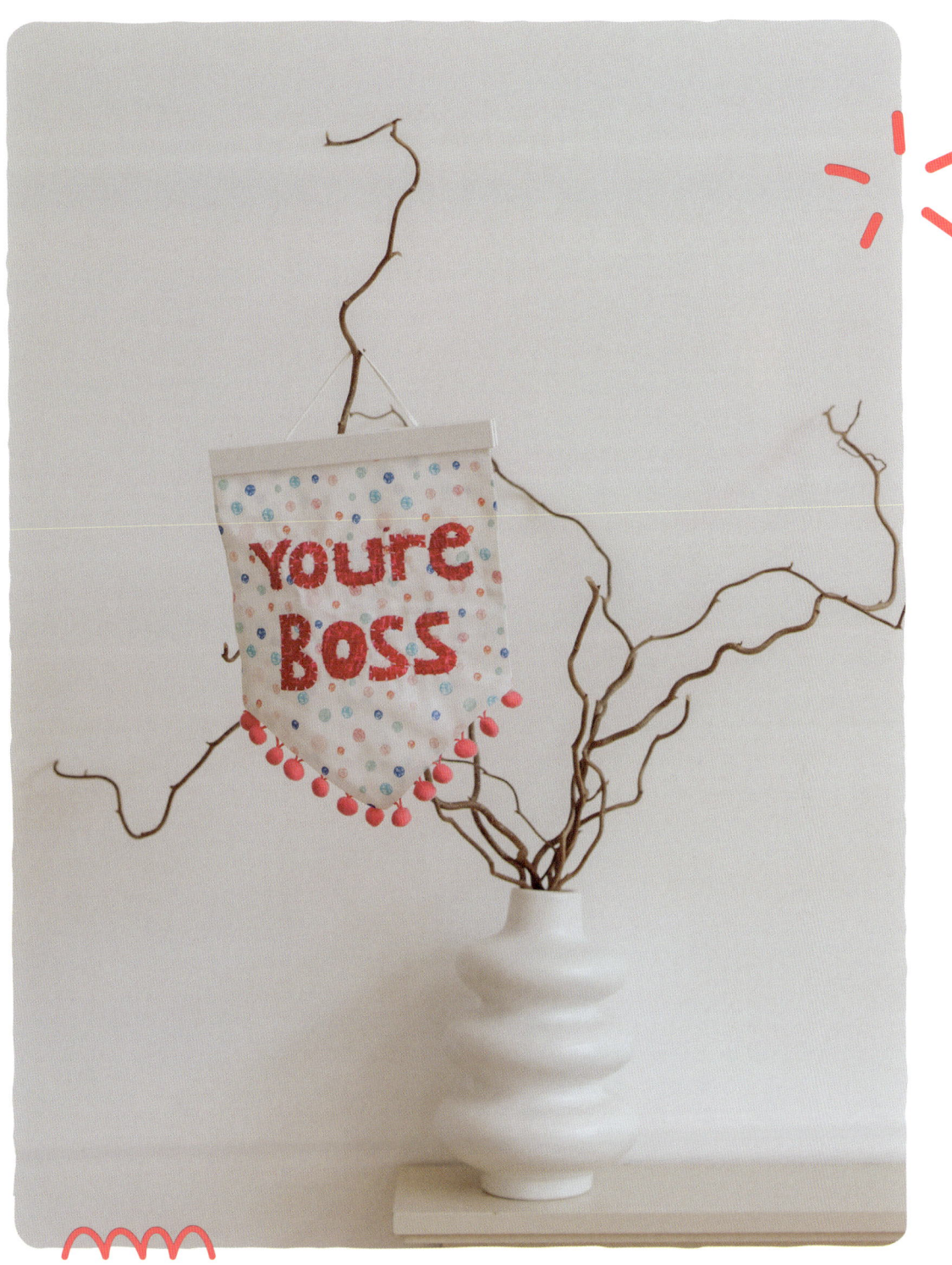

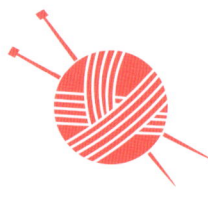

REWARDS OF KNITTING

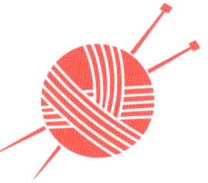

I love sitting at home on a winter's night, the rain pouring down outside, candles lit, fresh pjs and fluffy socks on, hot mug of tea in hand, wrapped up in a warm, snug blanket. Being warm and comfortable triggers our sense of safety, relieves tension and helps to shift us from a "fight or flight" (stressed) state to a "rest and digest" (relaxed) state. This shift is positively powerful for our wellbeing and state of mind.

As a textiles student I've always had a thing for texture and my house is filled with things like velvet chairs, knitted blankets and fluffy cushions. To me, different textures can create a cozy and comforting atmosphere and they help me to feel relaxed in my home.

I'm definitely a home bird.

My safe space

There is nowhere I feel safer than my bed. My bed is a big part of my life. You could say it's my comfort blanket. During my darkest days my bed was a place I never wanted to leave, and in the height of my depression I didn't leave it for days. It was the only place I wanted to be. I would sleep a lot. Sleep was an escape from my thoughts and emotions; if I was asleep,

I wouldn't be in pain.

When I'm overwhelmed I become extremely fatigued. My emotions take every tiny bit of energy I have. When I'm feeling like this, I embrace it and rest. Some may say I'm being dramatic but I've come to know myself and my body these days.

When I was depressed, sleeping, although a temporary relief, helped to regulate my mood. Unfortunately, you can't sleep off depression, so it's important we adopt behaviors and routines that can lift our mood on a more permanent basis – and that's where arts and crafts and creating as a mindfulness tool can come to the rescue; they certainly came to mine.

Today, my bed is the place I look forward to returning to at the end of the day. I'm really lucky that I'm a good sleeper; I'm actually known as Sleeping Beauty among my friends (I'll take it!). To be honest, I think it runs in the family because my mum is a very good sleeper and Sean was too. Actually, my mum spends more time getting her "beauty sleep" than she does awake!

Sleep is crucial for our overall health and wellbeing. A good night's sleep allows the body to rest and repair, supports brain function and enhances memory, boosts and regulates our mood and is essential for maintaining emotional resilience. Good news for my mum and me then!

My nan and her knitting

There are other activities that have been proven to have repairing and restoring benefits on our minds similar to sleep, and knitting is one of them. Knitting is a meditative activity. The repetitive motions can have a calming and relaxing effect on our mind and body, helping us to unwind and destress.

I remember my nan knitted a lot, especially when she was stressed. I'm not sure if she was aware of this, as we did not speak about it, but we all noticed she would pick up her needles whenever she needed to calm down – and with our family that was pretty regularly. My nan had four children, my mum, her sister and two brothers. My mum's brothers and sisters tested her, to say the least. But

when we lost Sean, she, like the rest of us, was heartbroken, not only for the loss of Sean but for my mum and me. My nan knitted continuous rows over and over and over; in fact, I'm not sure she even knew how to cast off. She always said she was knitting a scarf, but it was more of an art installation than a scarf! The huge mound of knitting was quite powerful to see, a true indication of just how stressed she must have been.

My mum knits for a similar reason but she always knits the same ball of wool. She knits until her ball of wool runs out, then she unravels all the knitting and starts again.

Knitting can be so rewarding. It offers a creative outlet, a sense of purpose, and a way to connect with others while creating beautiful and functional handmade items, items that fill us with joy and comfort. If you love knitting and want to meet new people, then knitting groups are popping up everywhere, so I'm sure there will be one close to you. Knitting groups are great for developing your skills. I could do with going to a class or two. A little like my nan, I generally knit pretty simple designs – scarves, blankets, fingerless mittens … anything that involves straight lines. I would love to be able to make those cute knitted dolls or those fab yarn bombings that cover the top of post boxes. But I have upped my game when it comes to knitting blankets …

Let's talk arm knitting!

CHUNKY-KNIT BLANKET

Once you've made one of these blankets, you will be making more, and if someone sees it … you will be making them for ever. It's just as well it's a therapeutic process!

We are going to create a cozy chunky-knit blanket, a satisfying project to make by hand. However, we're going to turn traditional knitting on its head and do something a little trendy … arm knitting! It is perfect for beginners and it's super effective.

No needles required!

YOU WILL NEED

★ **Chunky yarn** (such as wool or acrylic) – for a small 75cm x 125cm/30in x 50in blanket, use 2.7kg/6lb of yarn; for a large 1m x 1.5m/40in x 60in blanket use 3.6kg/8lbs of yarn

★ **Scissors**

NOTE: Working yarn is the yarn connected to the source.

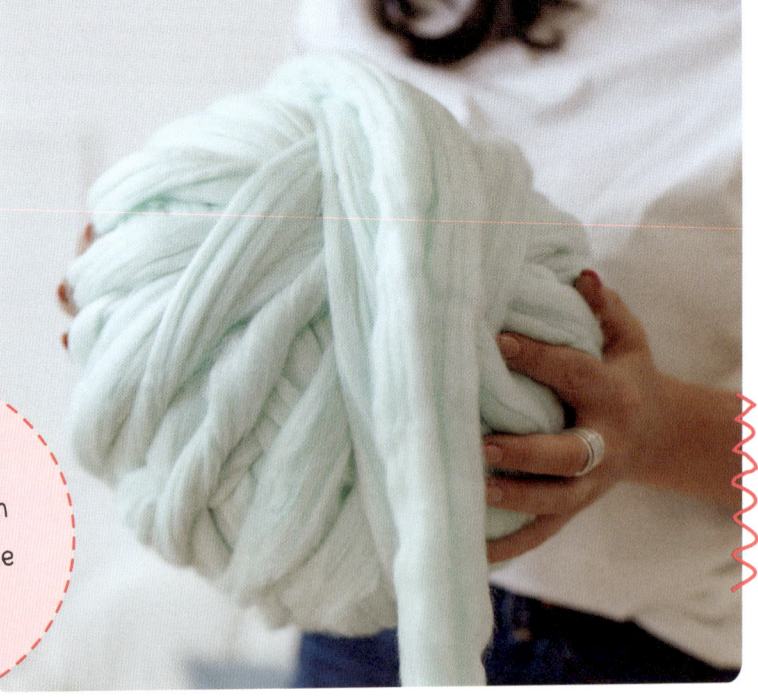

HOW TO MAKE A CHUNKY-KNIT BLANKET

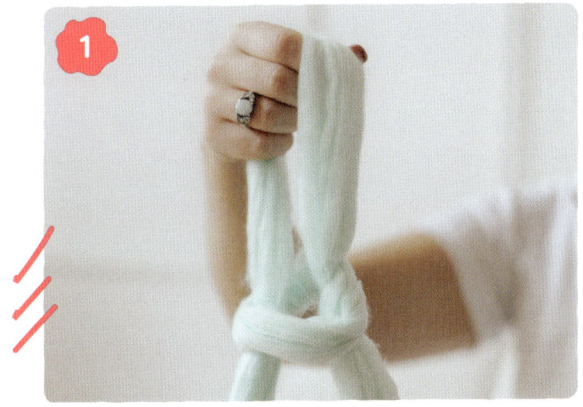

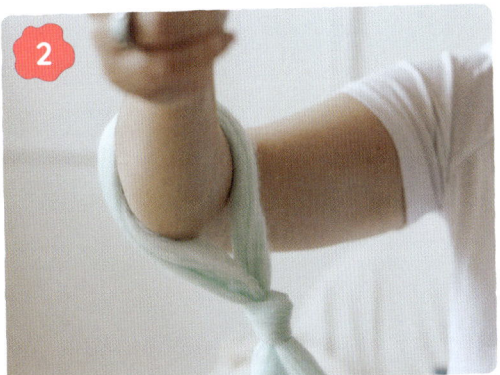

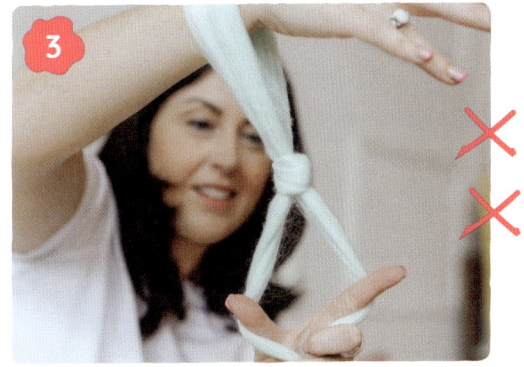

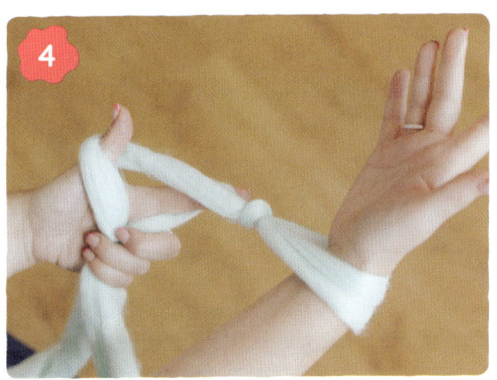

1. Measure out 2.5–3m/8–10 feet of wool and create a slip knot. This is essentially your first stitch.

2. Put the loop of the slip knot around your right wrist.

3. To begin your blanket, cast on your first row of stitches. To do so, take both the working yarn and the tail yarn in your left hand. Part the strands with your index finger and thumb.

4. Slip your hand (holding the slip knot) under the loop made on your opposite hand's thumb.

5. Cast the stitch onto your hand; you have cast on your first stitch.

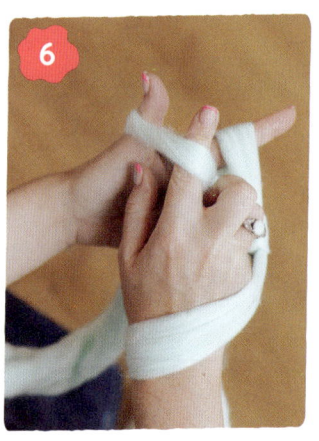
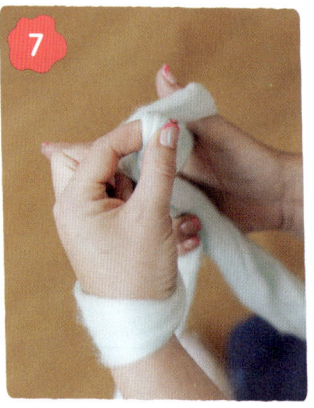
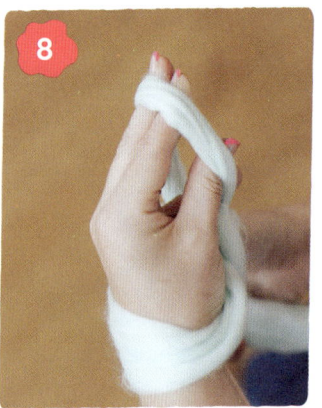
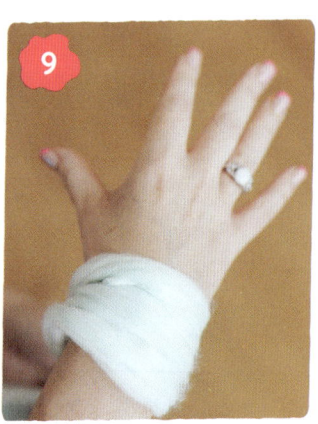

6. With the index finger of your working hand (the arm with the stitches), go under the tail yarn.

7. Then with your index finger and thumb, pick up the working yarn wrapped around your index finger.

8. Create a loop with the yarn over your right hand.

9. Slip the loop over your wrist. Congratulations, you have a stitch!!

10. Repeat this stage until you have cast a row of stitches. Use a loose tension and leave some wiggle room in each stitch.

11. This row of stitches will form the width of your blanket. Between 13 and 18 stitches is good for a medium-sized blanket.

12. Now we will knit the body of the blanket.

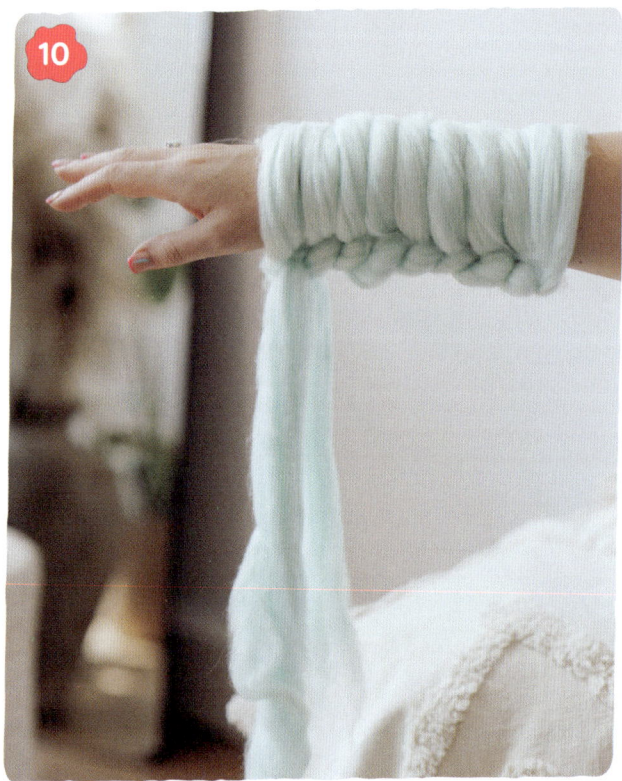

13. Holding the working yarn in your right hand, take the last stitch from your arm and pull it over and off your hand. This will form a loop, which will be your new stitch. Place this on your opposite arm.

14. Repeat this step for each of the stitches, moving all stitches from one arm to the other.

15. Tighten your stitches as you go, not too tight, but not too loose.

16. Continue this process by knitting your stitches and moving your stitches from one arm to the other. Continue arm knitting until you have around 5m/16 feet of yarn left.

17. You now need to cast off to ensure that your stitches don't unravel (see diagram overleaf). To do so, knit TWO stitches onto your opposite arm just like before.

18. Take the first of the two stitches and pull it over the second stitch and tighten. Knit one more stitch so you have TWO stitches on your arm again. Then again take the first of the two stitches and pull it over the second stitch and tighten.

19. Repeat until you're down to one stitch on your arm. Then cut your yarn about 1 metre/ 3 feet away from the blanket.

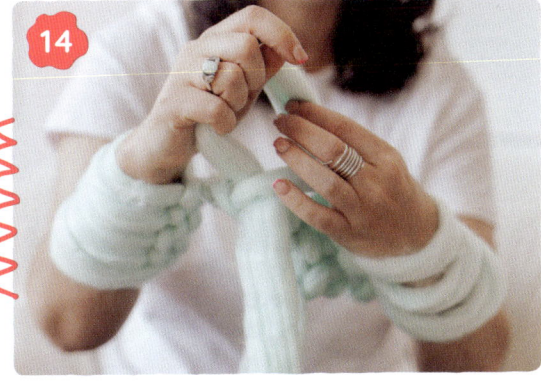

TIP: If you run out of yarn at any point and need to add more, simply tie the end of your yarn to a new ball of yarn in a tight knot.

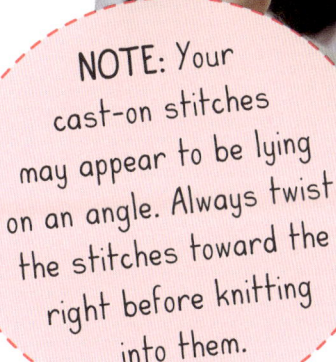

NOTE: Your cast-on stitches may appear to be lying on an angle. Always twist the stitches toward the right before knitting into them.

20. Pull the loose yarn through your last stitch and knot to secure the end of your blanket.

21. Go through your blanket gently, pulling out your stitches to stretch them out.

22. You now have your cast-on tail and your cast-off tail to tidy. Simply weave the tail strands of yarn through some of your previous stitches and then tie your tail yarn to one of your stitches with a tight knot. Trim off the excess.

⊕ Once you've completed these steps, your chunky-knit blanket is ready for those winter nights! Cozy up and relax.

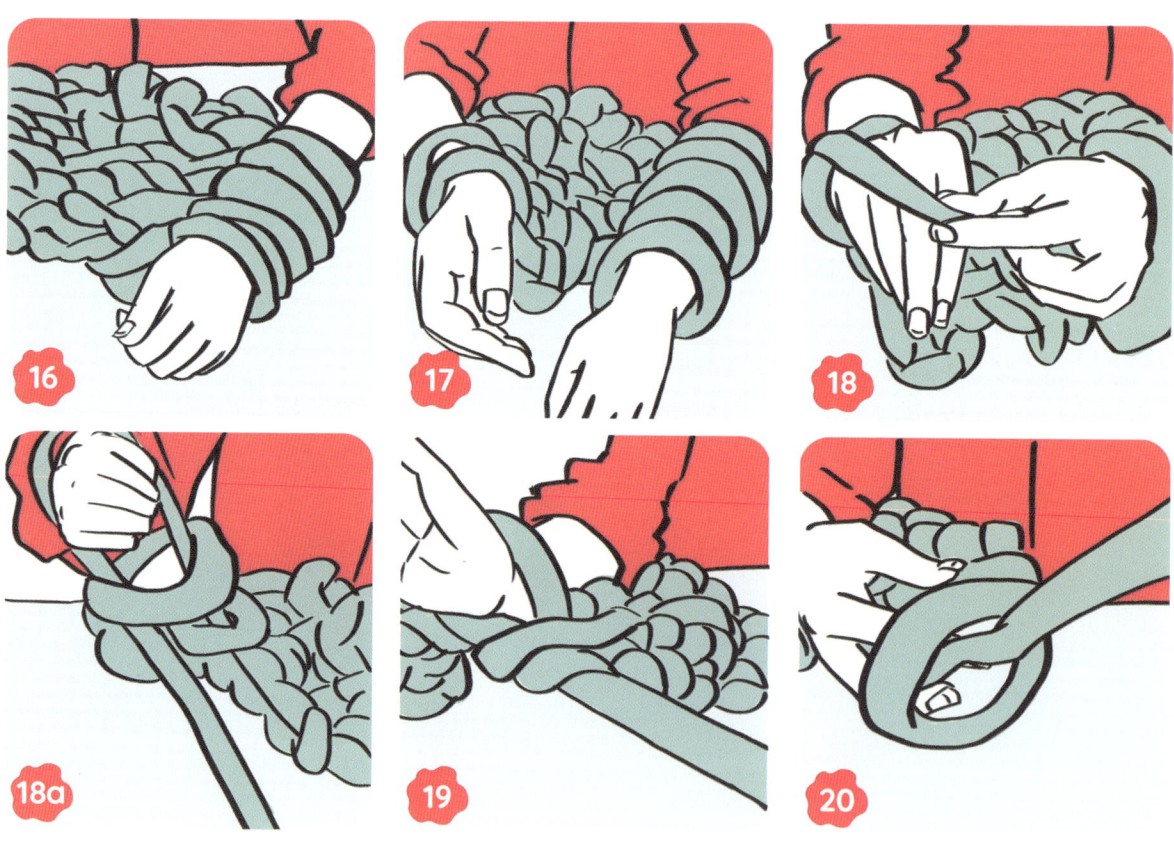

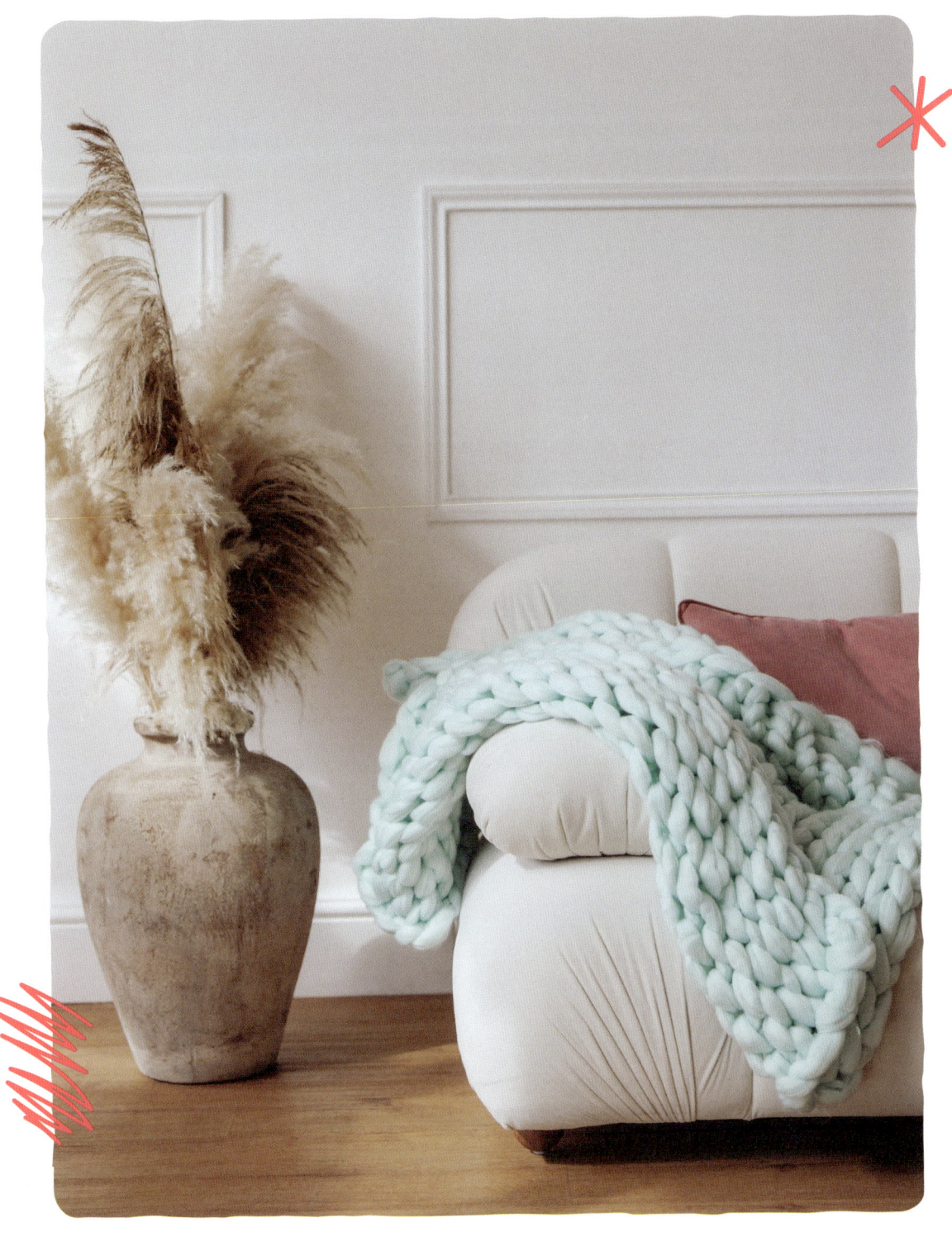

MAKING

WITH

MEMORIES

I cherish my memories, the good and the bad. Our memories are the most precious things we own, they are ours alone and nobody can take them away from us.

My most valuable memories are of my brother. I'm now unable to make new memories with him, which makes me hold the memories I have so very dearly. Losing Sean has shaped who I am. I'm sure I think about him more now than I would if he was still with me.

I try to celebrate Sean and his memory whenever I can, and crafting is a great way to do that. In fact, I use art to celebrate my memories and the special times I have had with all my loved ones, those that have passed and those that are still here. I use my memories as a constant source of inspiration for my art and craft projects. This often leads to deeply personal and meaningful projects.

I think about my childhood and in particular Sean a lot when crafting. The process of creating allows me to remember, and reliving these memories allows Sean to be alive in my mind. This, combined with the created tribute, is a powerful and special experience.

I use what I have – photographs, memorabilia, clothing, furniture, books … anything that sparks joy and honours my memories of my loved ones. Here I've included some of my favourite crafting projects that I've made with my memories. I hope it inspires you to create special keepsakes that can be cherished for years to come.

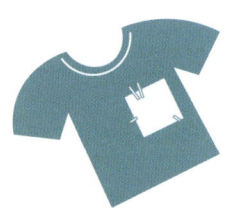
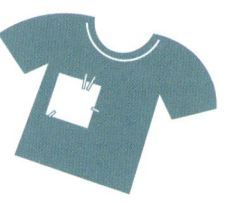

CRAFTING WITH CLOTHING

When it comes to arts and crafts, you don't need expensive materials and tools to create with. I love to use what I have around me and I only buy new when it's absolutely necessary. Repurposing old clothing is simply great for crafting – you can create items and gifts that have meanings and memories.

We all need a cuddle sometimes. There's nothing better than putting your arms around the person you love. Feel-good hormones flood our body, leaving us feeling happier, calmer and altogether more relaxed.

When you're feeling down, a big hug is often better than a thousand words. However, when your cuddle companion is no longer around, it's simply devastating. There were many nights I fell asleep wishing I could have one more cuddle from my little brother. Like most brothers and sisters, we argued and fought, but we always had a cuddle before going to bed.

Comfy clothes

After photographs, clothing is what most people keep to remember their loved ones. Clothes can hold so many stories and memories.

When we lost Sean, my mum struggled with what we should do with his things, in particular his clothes, and for a while we did nothing. His clothes sat in his drawers for months; his Liverpool football kit hung in his wardrobe, his karate kit sat unused and his Ninja Turtle pyjamas lay on the bottom of his bed exactly where he'd left them. They lay unwashed, as my mum was afraid that if she washed them we would lose his smell. I would occasionally give them a sniff and breathe in his aroma, a mix of chocolate buttons and Lynx Africa. Even at the age of nine Sean wanted to impress the ladies! As I held the soft cotton up against my face, tears filled my eyes, but I could see him.

Eventually, we packed Sean's things away. His empty bedroom became a constant reminder of his absence. My mum could not bear to part with his clothes, so she neatly folded them into storage boxes and stored them away. This is where they stayed, until I was studying for my master's.

The Wendy house

During my postgraduate studies, I did a lot of soul-searching and extensive research into art therapy, in particular art therapy for bereaved children. To conclude my research and complete my studies I needed to create a final piece of artwork. This is when Sean's clothes came out of the storage boxes – they would have a new purpose.

The Wendy house was a piece of art I created by hand-stitching together Sean's clothes, fabrics from our childhood and textiles printed with photos of our childhood. The Wendy house encapsulates both the joyful memory of my little brother and my emotions after his loss, and it celebrates the short time we spent together. The house is a place for special games and secret fantasy worlds, a place that puts a boundary between the child and the rest of the world, a place of safety and comfort, a space for reflection.

Creating this artwork became an important stage in my healing process. Sifting through Sean's clothes after almost 12 years, I was flooded with memories of him. I could envision him in these clothes and I remembered special

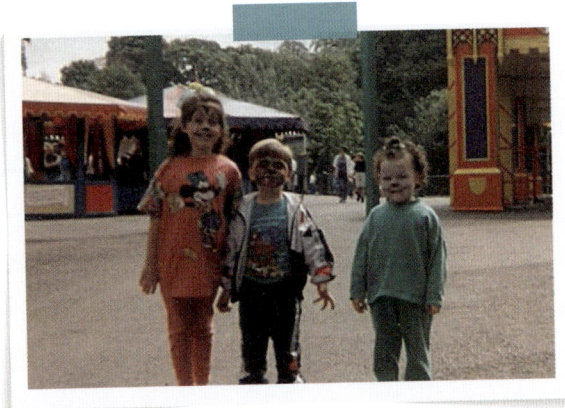

moments with each garment I came across, like his favourite pink T-shirt that he loved to wear on holiday because he thought it brought out his tan!

Hand-stitching the entire thing together allowed me to process the conflicting emotions that came up. The slow, repetitive movement of pulling a needle and thread through the garments became almost meditative. I shed many tears while constructing the house and released a lot of built-up emotion and frozen grief.

Sewing is recognized as an effective way to combat stress and depression. It's the repetitive flow that comes with needlework that allows you to centre yourself. Both your mind and body can fully relax while your hands create. It's here that the process becomes as much the art form as the created outcome.

Reusing your loved ones' clothes for a sewing project is a great way to keep their memories alive. You can create unique items to be cherished.

COMFORTING CUSHION

Here we're going to create a cushion, the perfect comforter for those moments when you just need a cuddle, and it's a great starting point if you're a sewing beginner.

This is a great activity to reuse old clothing. You might want to use that lucky top that no longer fits, the baby's first babygrow or your school-leaver's shirt that's covered in the signatures of your classmates. Regardless of what memories you're creating from, this repurposing craft is a fun and creative way to keep your hands busy, focus your mind and upcycle your preloved clothing.

The little details such as the seams, buttons, pockets and labels add that something extra to a project that you just wouldn't get with fabric off the roll.

If you're using clothes belonging to a loved one, this could be a daunting task. I would recommend sorting through old clothing separately to this task and put aside the items you would like to use. You may need some time to process the emotions that come up from sorting through the old belongings.

Your cushion can be made up of small pieces of fabric patched together or larger pieces such as a shirt or jumper – or maybe one side could be patched and the other made from a larger piece.

YOU WILL NEED

★ **2 pieces of fabric** – for the front and back of the cushion. The amount of fabric needed depends on the cushion size. The fabric is cut exactly the same size as the cushion. My cushion is 40cm x 40cm (16in x 16in), so both pieces of my fabric are cut 40cm x 40cm (16in x 16in). You could use a paper template the exact size of the cushion to help.

★ Pins

★ **Embroidery sewing needle** – an embroidery needle is perfect for this project, as it has a bigger eyelet, allowing for thicker thread. You could use a sewing machine for this activity, but I find hand-sewing much more therapeutic

★ **Thread** – I like to use embroidery threads in contrasting colours to my fabrics because I like to see the stitching. You may want to use thread the same colour as your fabrics

★ **Sharp fabric scissors**

★ **Iron**

★ **Cushion** – if you're anything like me, you will have plenty you can reuse from around the house. If not, you can buy cushion inners in a variety of shapes and sizes from a range of stores or online.

HOW TO CREATE A COMFORTING CUSHION

1. Cut out your two pieces of fabric. If you're using smaller patches of fabric, you will need to stitch them together first.

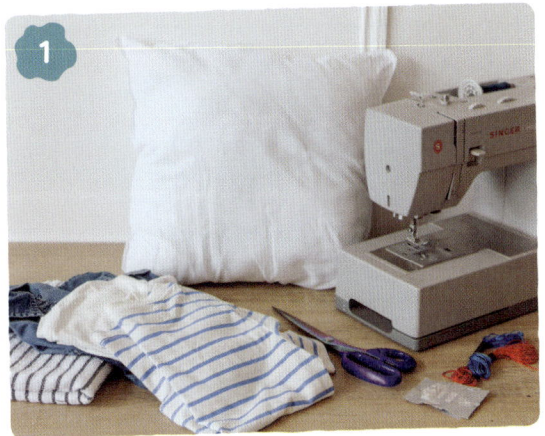

2. Pin the pieces of fabric together – you want the "wrong" sides facing outwards and the sides that will become the outside of the cushion facing inwards (i.e. it's inside out). Leave the bottom side of the cover open so that the pillow can be inserted later.

3. Thread your needle (the most fiddly part!). Start hand-sewing the fabrics together using a simple running stitch, leaving a 2cm border around the edge.

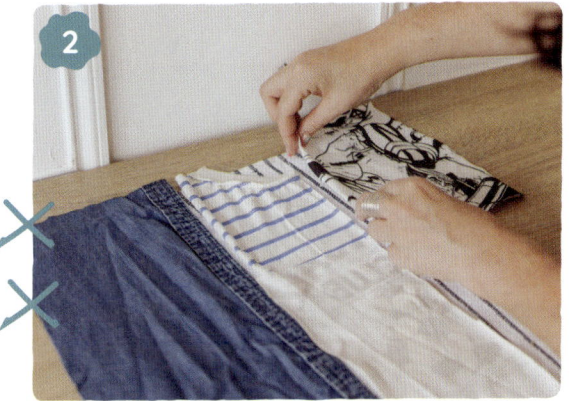

4. Sew all the way around three sides of the pillow, leaving the bottom side open.

Running stitch — — — — —

5. Knot your thread by taking a small piece of fabric right next to where your thread is. Pull your needle and thread through, but not all the way, leaving a small loop of thread. Put your needle through the loop and pull through. Repeat.

6. Snip the fabric on the four corners, making sure not to cut your stitches.

7. Turn your cushion cover inside out, so that it's now right side out. Now's the time to iron your cover.

8. Insert your cushion and pin the bottom side of the cover closed.

9. Hand-sew the pillow closed using a ladder stitch, folding in the edge of your fabric as you go to create a neater seam. You could continue to use a running stitch but I find a ladder stitch neater for this finished edge.

⊕ A cushion is a great introduction to creating with your preloved clothing. Making cushions from clothes belonging to a family member is a meaningful way to honour their memory and create keepsakes that will be treasured for years to come.

There are so many fabulous and super-easy projects to make use of preloved clothing, such as scrap bags and scrap lampshades (see pages 84 and 88), decorative weaving (see page 112) and even an upholstered chair (see page 156).

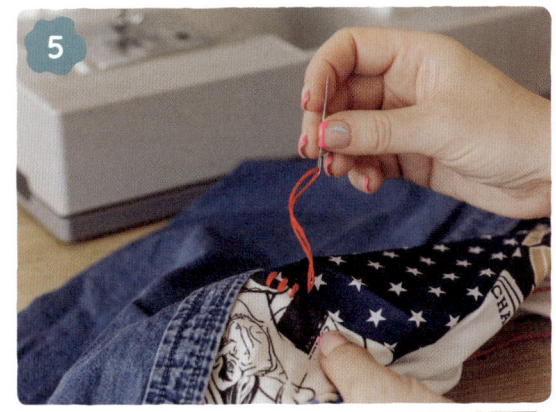

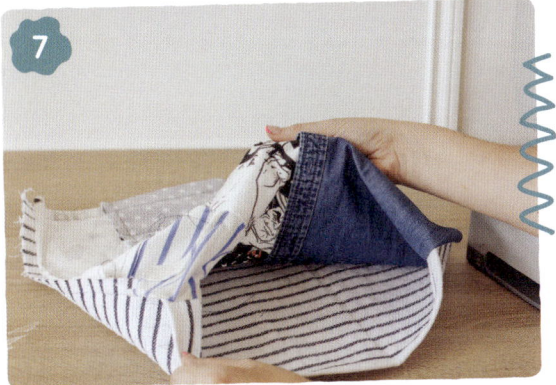

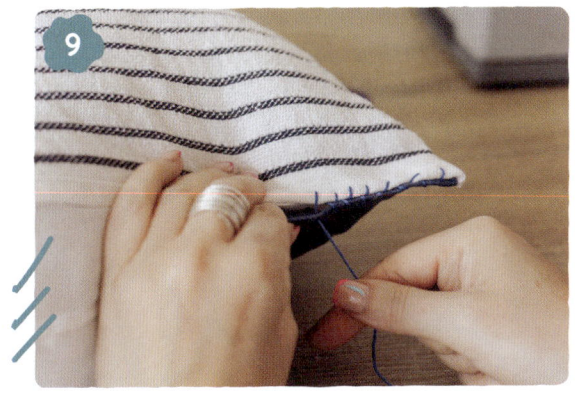

Ladder stitch |||||||||||||||||||||||||||||

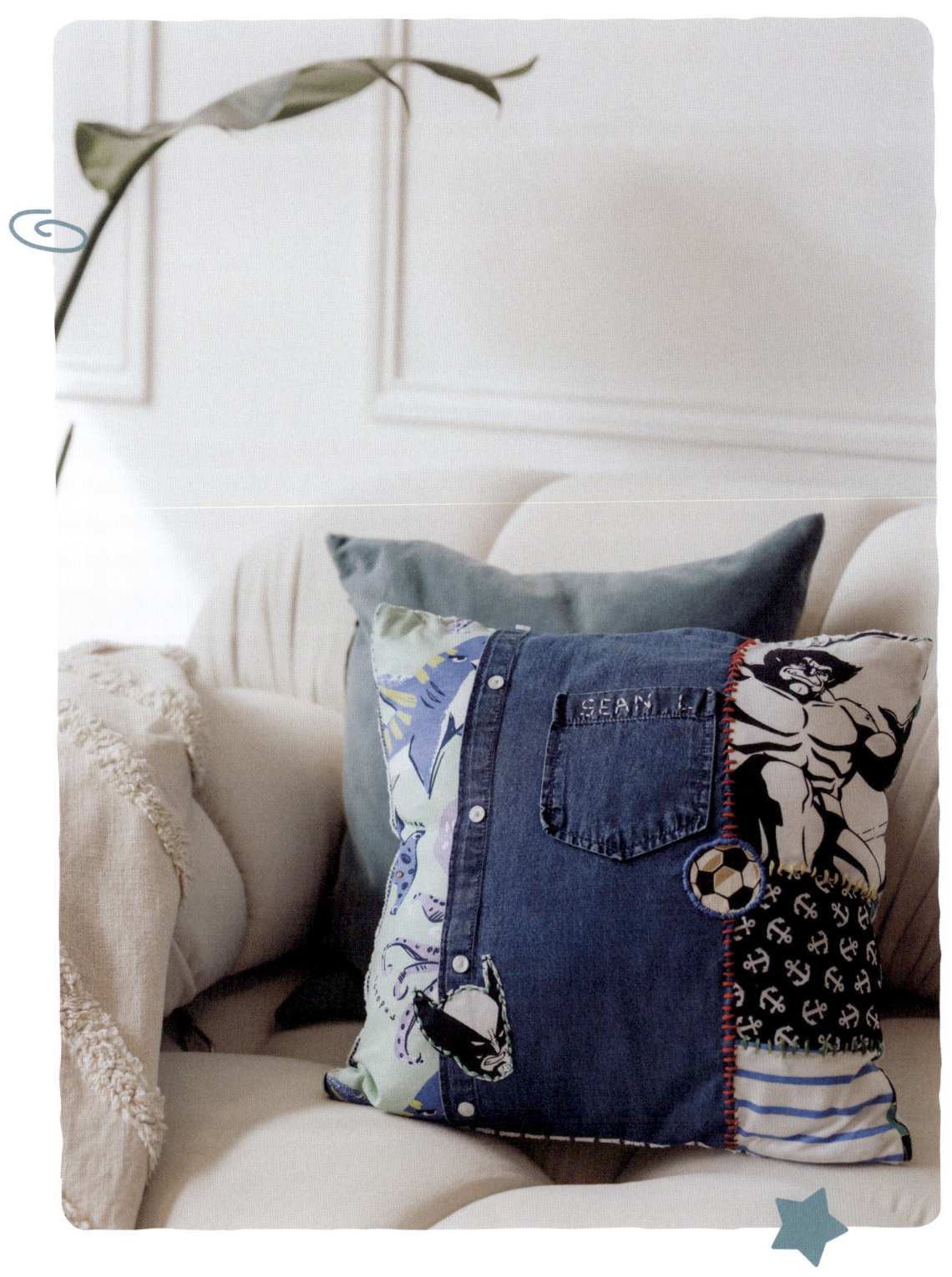

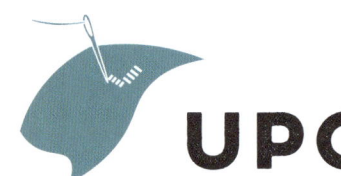

UPCYCLING SCRAP FABRICS

You are probably starting to realize that I throw nothing away! As I've said, repurposing old clothing is great for craft projects; add old tea towels, tired bedsheets, unwanted curtains and fabric scraps to the mix and you'll have a constant supply of materials ready for crafting action. This is a clever way to reduce the environmental impact of the clothing and textile industry, which is one of the largest polluting industries in the world.

My mum is an absolute whizz on the sewing machine. She loves making cushions and curtains and even made clothes for Sean and me when we were growing up.

I have a vivid memory of her sitting at the sewing machine at the kitchen table one Christmas Eve. I must have been about nine, which would have made Sean six. We'd had our Christmas bath and were in bed in our new Christmas pyjamas, giddy with excitement for the arrival of Father Christmas.

We had been in bed for a while but I was too excited to sleep. I was thinking about all the wonderful presents I would receive the next day. (I was a good girl so I always got lots of presents.) While I lay there playing out Christmas morning in my head, I heard the humming of the sewing machine coming from downstairs. Curious, I got out of bed and sat at the top of the stairs. I wondered why I could hear the sewing machine on Christmas Eve in what felt like the middle of the night. Was it Father Christmas? Had he caught his jacket on his sleigh and was doing a quick repair?

I crept down the stairs and peered around the kitchen door, only to find my mum, sat at the machine in her Christmas pyjamas. Oblivious to the fact I was there, she continued to stitch a gold ribbon to a pair of black trousers – trousers that looked remarkably similar to the Michael Jackson trousers Sean had on his Christmas list. This was the moment I found out that my mum was working for Father Christmas! Of all the evenings for this revelation!

Family upcycling

With my mum a machinist, my nan a keen knitter and my grandad painting and drawing, I grew up around lots of arts and crafts. These sorts of activities were a big part of our lives. They weren't hobbies as such and certainly not professions, just something they did.

They didn't have expensive tools and materials; they used what they had. Anything and everything was potential material. This hasn't changed; I've grown up constantly reusing and upcycling.

My grandad was also a keen gardener and always had such a beautiful well-kept garden. He loved to repurpose items for his garden; anything and everything became a plant pot, from the usual yogurt pots to washing-up bowls. However, his garden shed was something of a masterpiece, at least in my eyes, as it was made from scrap wood, old doors and windows.

Making cushions and curtains was Mum's thing. It was an easy way to transform our home without having to redecorate. I loved to collect the scrap fabrics when she'd finished her creations. At the time I never knew exactly what I would use them for but I always knew they would come in handy one day.

A very heavy bag

Fresh out of university, I was volunteering at the Alder Centre (the bereavement services at Alder Hey Children's Hospital), which provides support to anyone affected by the death of a child and is an incredibly valuable resource for families such as mine. While I was volunteering there, I worked alongside a counsellor called Jenny Mercer, and between the two of us we put together a resource for bereaved children.

The resource was an illustrated short story about a bear who had lost his special person. The bear was on a journey and carried with him a very heavy bag. This bag was filled with heavy stones, each stone representing his feelings – sadness, anger, anxiety and fear. While on his journey, the bear took regular breaks to rest, and at each stop he took a stone out of his backpack and tackled the emotion associated with it. The bear ended his journey with a much lighter bag, having worked through his heavy emotions and lightened his initially heavy load.

Just like the bear, we all carry our emotions around with us. When they become too heavy, it's important we express them. My bag can often feel too heavy to carry. When it does, I try to allow myself time to rest. However, I often find it difficult to relax and switch off, so giving myself tasks such as crafting can keep my hands busy while giving my mind a much-needed break.

So, while we are on the subject of bags, let's make one.

SCRAP BAG

This book is evidence that I use up all my collected preloved treasures. I see purpose, a story and quite often sentiment in everything. Here we're going to create a unique bag using scrap fabrics. If you are after a craft that requires little to no concentration, then this is the one for you. The repetitive action is almost meditative and can help you to unwind – it's mindful relaxation!

This simple project is perfect for using up any crafting offcuts, old bedsheets or even old tea towels, bits of fabric that are all too often not good enough for larger projects. It's also a great way to use up old clothes that you've outgrown or damaged or possibly those of a loved one that you don't want to part with. Transform them into something you can carry around with you every day.

I use torn fabrics in a lot of my crafts, and I find tearing the fabric is a therapeutic activity in itself. Maybe it's the force required that provides an instant release of energy, or maybe it's the sound ... If you're into your ASMR, this is a great one!

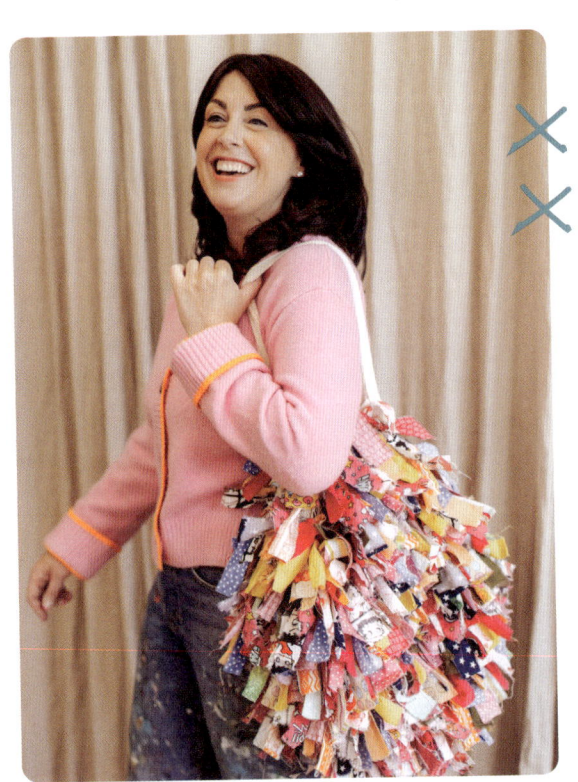

YOU WILL NEED

★ **Scrap fabrics** or **old clothes**

★ **Scissors**

★ **A string bag**

HOW TO CREATE A SCRAP BAG

1. Tear or cut your fabrics into strips, 5cm x 20cm/2in x 8in approximately. But don't worry too much about the exact measurements. You will need a lot of strips to make your bag big and fluffy like mine, anywhere between 200 and 400 strips!

2. Take the fabric strips and one by one tie them to the strings of the bag with knots.

⊕ And that is it! This is such a simple project, but it can take time. My bag took three hours to complete, but I'm sure you'll agree it was well worth it. The bag looks great and I've given myself three full hours to relax, unwind and take a break.

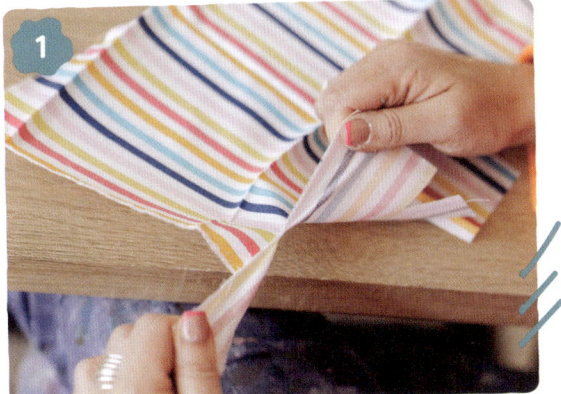

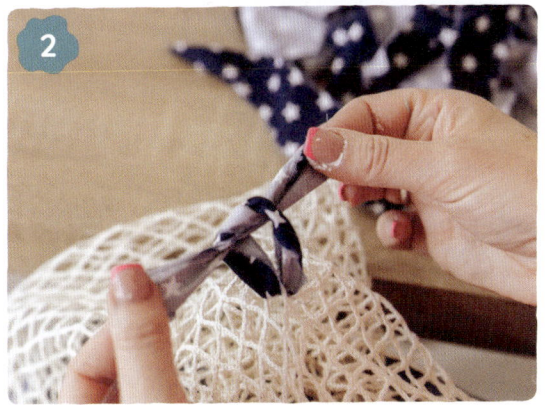

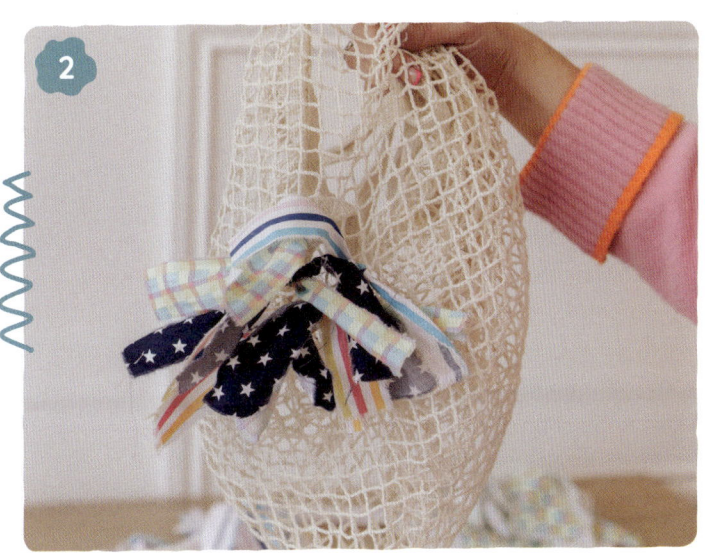

LIGHT UP YOUR LIFE

Lighting can enhance our mood, productivity and overall wellbeing and can influence our energy levels and even our sleep patterns. It's worth giving some thought to how you light your home and in particular your creative space. It can be a great opportunity to personalize this space with one-of-a-kind upcycling projects – you might as well have some fun with it and make something uniquely yours.

Looking back on my darker times, dark is exactly what they were … I would spend hours in dark rooms, sleeping my days away, unable to face daylight. It felt like my life had no joy, happiness or hope. It was as if my light had gone out.

As my depression lifted, I allowed more light into my life; I was able to see more clearly what I had around me, the love of my family and the support of my friends being the most important.

Today I try to surround myself with as much light as possible. Light allows us to see a little clearer and provides even the smallest glimmer of hope.

Now, I love my home to be filled with light. I have a mixture of standing lamps, table lamps, desk lamps large and small, spotlights, fairy lights and candlelight. Among them are many of my own projects, lamps that I have fashioned out of cups and saucers, bottles and even reels of cotton, handpainted lampshades that I mix and match on painted and vintage bases and ceiling lights filled with feathers.

Lighting and mental health

I find lighting sets the mood for the space. In my home I've opted for welcoming, comfortable and warm with lots of natural light. My dark days are over.

Here's a little rundown of how different types of lighting can affect us, which is something worth considering for your creative space and overall mental health.

Exposure to natural light during the day improves mood and energy levels. Sunlight boosts the production of serotonin, making us feel calmer and happier, which is probably why we are all a little grumpy here in England in the winter – we rarely see the sun!

Bright light can enhance alertness and concentration, which is worth considering when choosing your space to create. A well-lit area can be particularly beneficial when you need to focus and be productive.

Warm lighting (my favourite) creates a cozy and relaxing atmosphere. It can help reduce stress and create a sense of comfort, making it ideal for living rooms and bedrooms. Dim lighting creates a more intimate and relaxing environment, which can be beneficial for unwinding before bed.

Blue light exposure, especially from screens such as laptops and smartphones, can disrupt sleep patterns if used in the evening. So try your best to put the phone away at least one hour before bed to get a good night's sleep.

The *Find It, Fix It, Flog It* team often get joked about for the amount of lamps we make on the show. We've transformed telephones, petrol cans, tree trunks, bird boxes and hair dryers into lighting! But all jokes aside, upcycling and repurposing items into lighting leads to fabulous transformations. I'm a sucker for lighting and a huge fan of lamps big and small. My home is full of them, and now I'm about to add another ...

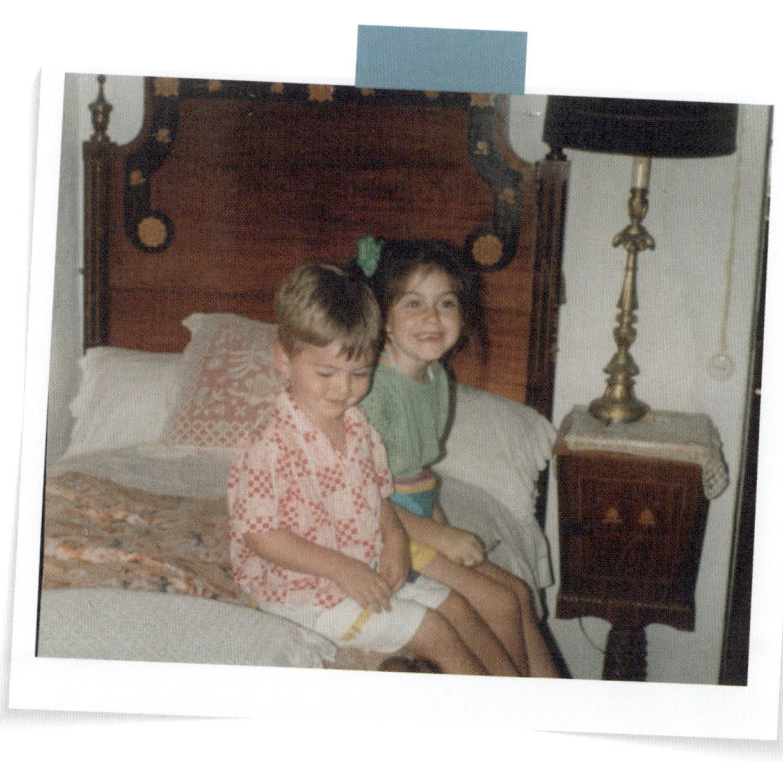

SCRAP LAMPSHADE

Considering what we now know about lighting and how it affects our mood, let's make a lampshade that will create a warm and comfortable space where we can unwind, relax and destress.

Scrap lampshades are a great way to use up scraps of fabric. I'm using lots of offcuts of fabrics from previous projects, but you could use anything you can get your hands on – old curtains, tea towels and bedding are ideal for this. Old clothes are great for lampshades too; shirts with buttons or pockets add character, and embroidered details always look super cute – and how lovely would it be to have the clothing of your loved one light up your room.

Bear in mind the fabric, as we want to let light through the shade, so heavy wools and dense fabrics may not work for this. But that certainly doesn't mean they won't come in handy for other projects.

I'm making my lampshade from scratch, but you could easily upcycle an old or tired lampshade to create the same look. This method on an old-fashioned bell lampshade would look amazing. Ohh, actually, I must add that to my to-do list!

YOU WILL NEED

★ **Scrap fabrics** – different colours and patterns make for a more quirky shade. I've chosen strips approximately 5cm/2in wide, the length will depend on the size of your shade. For a smaller lampshade you will need around 20 strips, 40 for a standard ceiling shade and up to 150 for a bell shade.

★ **A lampshade kit** – everything you need to make a lampshade. You can buy them online and in some craft stores in a variety of shapes and sizes. I've gone for a 25cm/10in drum lampshade to fit my small table lamp.

TOP TIP: Make sure the "bulb" frame is in the correct place, depending on how you're hanging your lampshade.

If you don't plan on making lampshades regularly, then a kit is ideal for you. If, however, you are planning on making lampshades regularly or maybe a large batch for gifts, then you can buy all of the materials separately.

To purchase materials separately you will need:

★ **Self-adhesive lampshade panel** – you can buy this on the roll and cut to size depending on the size of the lampshade you are making

★ **Lampshade frames** – these come in a variety of sizes

★ **Binding tape**

★ **Finishing tool**

★ **Fabric glue**

HOW TO MAKE A SCRAP LAMPSHADE

1. Start by tearing or cutting your scrap fabrics into strips. Make sure they are long enough to cover your lampshade panel vertically. Don't worry if they are a little longer than your lampshade – we can trim to size once they are all in place. I find tearing the fabric into strips is a therapeutic activity in itself!

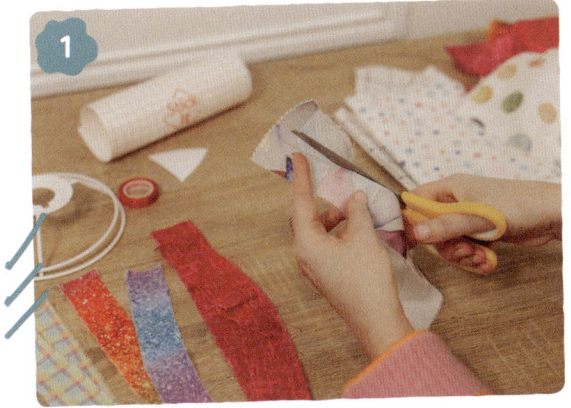

2. Lay out the self-adhesive panel and peel back the paper (you may need to weigh down the edges with weights)

3. Lay your fabric strips over the adhesive panel, pressing each down securely as you go.

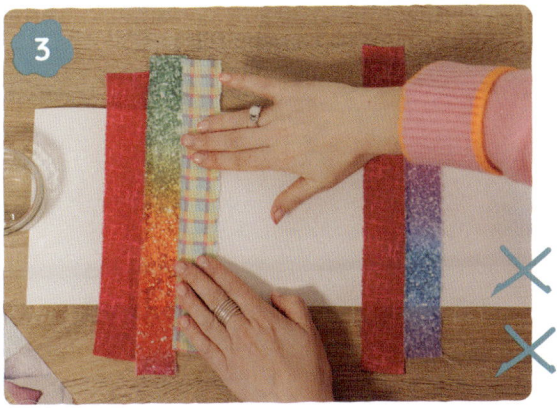

4. Once the panel is filled with your fabric strips, trim the lengths of fabric to the size of the panel.

5. Snap back the top and bottom edges of the panel until they break. Carefully peel back the edges from the backing panel, trying to avoid the fabric peeling away from the panel. You can now put this to one side for the moment.

6. Using the double-sided binding tape, tape around the circumference of the two frame pieces. Fold the tape around the frame and remove the tape backing.

7. This is where a third arm would come in handy. Lay the lampshade panel out flat, wrong side up (using weights to keep it flat if needed) and place the two frames on either side of the lampshade panel.

8. Roll the frames along the edges of the panel until you reach the end, sticking the frame to the fabric as you go. It's starting to take shape!

9. Use the finishing tool to tuck in the fabric underneath the frame to neaten the edges. Snip a line where the lightbulb support part of the frame is, so that the fabric can be wrapped around this area.

10. You may need to use fabric glue to secure the ends of the lampshade panel. Once the glue is dry, the lampshade is then ready to be used!

We don't always want to be standing in the spotlight, but even when you want to hide yourself away, add a little light to your day by switching on your lamp ... You will see a little clearer, I promise.

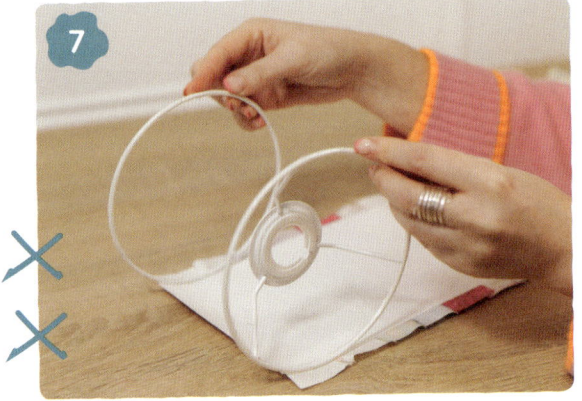

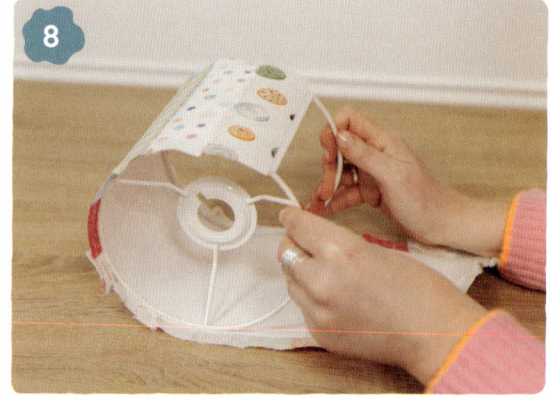

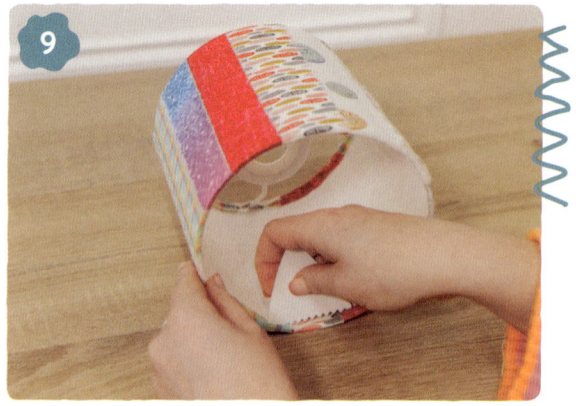

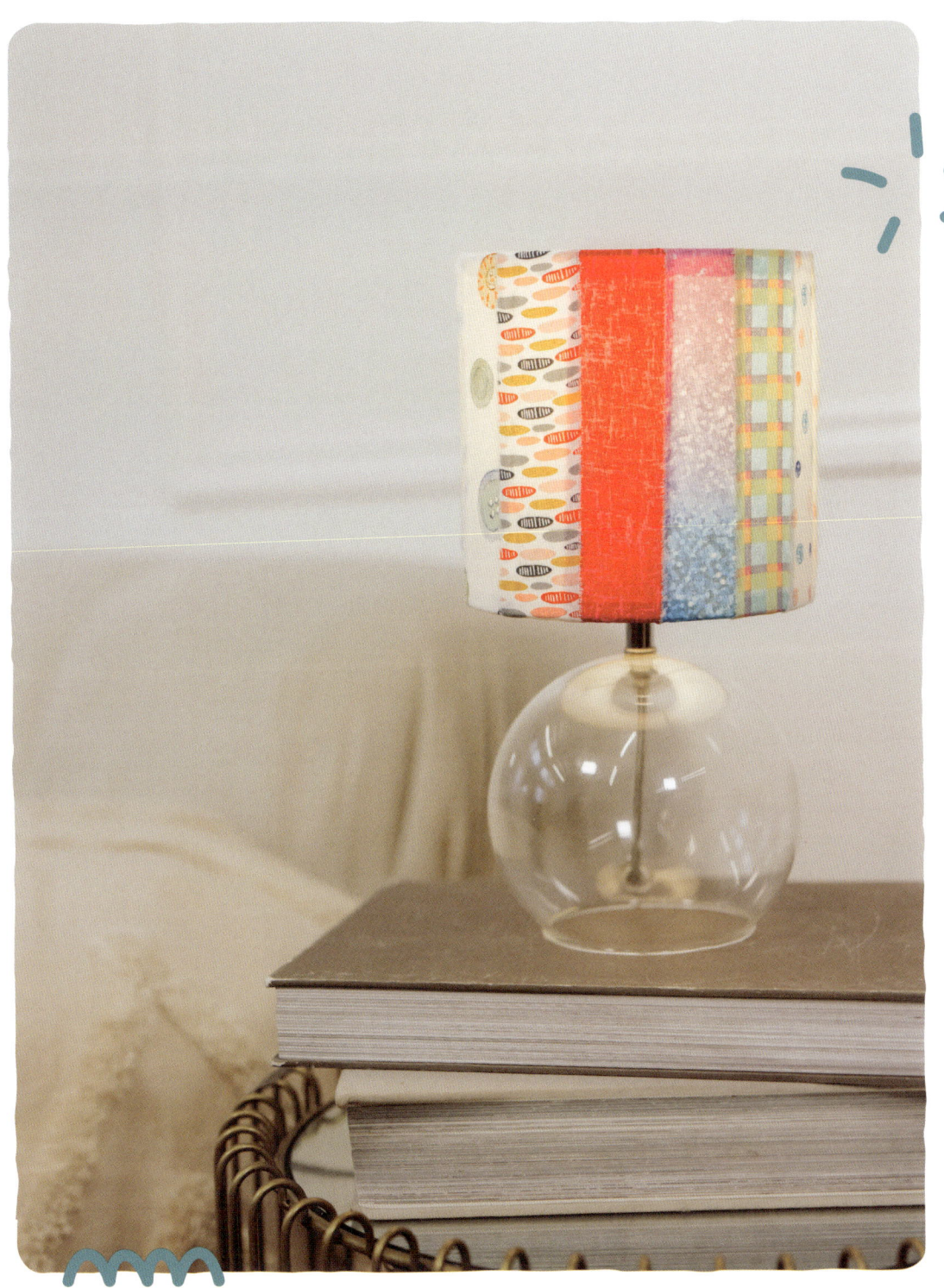

REVAMPING WITH STENCILS

Upcycling is a great way to inject character into our homes. Revamped one-of-a-kind items make for great statement pieces. I think it's important that our home reflects our personality, as this allows us to truly relax and be ourselves when we are in it. This is hugely important for our emotional development and mental health.

I recently worked with a children's home who offer a home to children temporarily. The children have very few belongings and are given a room that many other children have used before them. I worked with the children when they arrived at the home to create items for their rooms that represented who they are, their interests and passions – items that allowed them to make their mark on their space, make their room their own. For the children, having their own space with their own belongings is hugely valuable; it gives them a sense of belonging which boosts confidence and their emotional wellbeing.

These children don't have a lot of memorabilia to create with, so I love that I'm creating new memories with them. Who knows where the furniture will end up in the future? A bedside cabinet painted now could end up in

their granddaughter's bedroom years into the future.

Decorating my home

My house is an extension of me; it's full of colour, half-finished projects and lots of photographs. At the moment I rent but I do dream of owning my home one day. There's just the small matter of saving up for a deposit.

When it comes to decorating my home, my landlord is pretty flexible and he has said I can do whatever I like and make it my own. But I am still very conscious that it's not my house. So I do what I can to add personality and character without compromising it. Saying that, I have wallpapered most rooms in floral wallpaper and the remaining walls are painted pink, I've added stencils to the bathroom tiles and even the patio flooring – but that's all reversible, of course!

My house is filled with my memories. I've got photos everywhere, my nan's nick-nacks out on display and Mum's old cushions and curtains when she changes her mind every couple of months. I do love a hand-me-down, I love to make use of something I know is being discarded. However, I also like to add my stamp, make my mark and visually add my chapter to the item's story. A great way of doing this is stencilling – it's the perfect way for me to add my personality to my mum's soft furnishings.

Dreams

When I was younger, I had big plans for myself. I had a timeline all laid out with milestones I wanted to reach. But here I am, 40 years old, not having reached any of them. Honestly, I'm ok with it,

I'm on a different path – maybe one that's been a little more challenging and less traditional than I had thought, but I wouldn't change any of it, it's made me who I am. Most days I like myself, I'm happy with who I am as a person. I believe I'm kind, passionate and loyal; I work hard and I'm doing the best I can to make my dreams come true. And I'm pretty confident they will.

One day I will own my house, but for now I'm in my rented home that I love and feel comfortable in. I took this house on as a way of escaping a relationship and it was the best move I ever made. I see it as my little sanctuary; I have grown and changed for the better within the safety of this house.

Regardless of whether your home is bought or rented, you can easily add your personality to it by upcycling. Upcycling isn't just for furniture, it's also great for transforming soft furnishings.

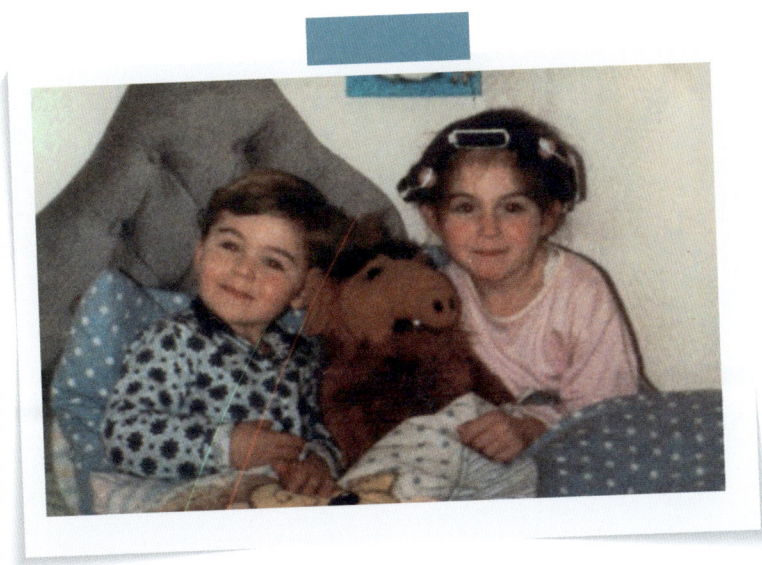

STENCILLED CURTAINS

I want to show you a pretty simple way to put your stamp on your home: revamping soft furnishings with stencils. Here we are using curtains. Stencils are a great way to transform something a little dull into something unique.

Stencils are used a lot in street art, and I'm here for it. I do love that graffiti style and the rebellious attitude of making your mark wherever you want. There may be a stigma associated with this but if it's good enough for Banksy then it's good enough for me.

Aside from the rebellious street art, stencils are a great way to reproduce a pattern, which makes them great for soft furnishings. Apparently they have been in use for 2,000 years. I wasn't around then

so I can't confirm this information, but it has come from a reliable source. Early stencils were used to replicate expensive fabrics; however, nowadays stencils have come into their own and are no longer used purely to imitate other work.

Stencilling is easy to do and once you've got to grips with the technique, there really is no stopping you. Like me, you'll find yourself collecting old fabrics, cushion covers, bedding and curtains for future stencilling projects.

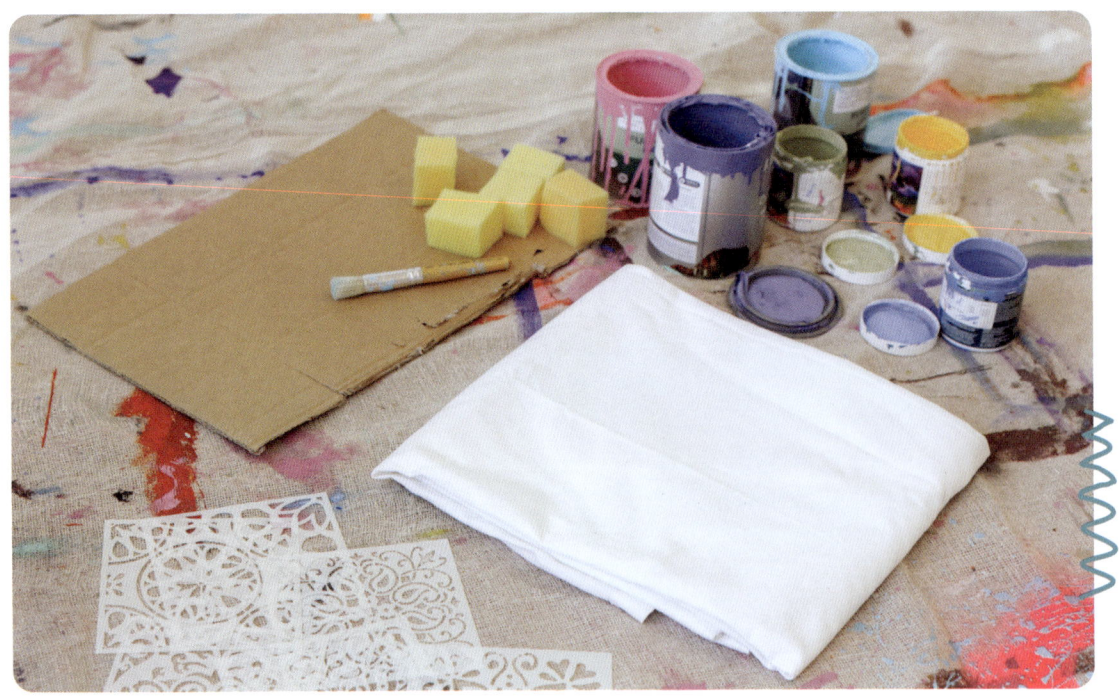

YOU WILL NEED

★ **Card** or **acetate** – or if you want to be a pro then you can get stencil film, but don't use paper, it's too thin

★ A Pencil for drawing

★ **Craft scalpel knife** or **scissors**

HOW TO MAKE A STENCIL

You can buy stencils online and in most craft and DIY stores, but sometimes you have a look in mind that you can't find the right stencil for, so in this instance, make your own! It's super easy, so let me show you how.

If you're a beginner to stencilling, I'd stick to the larger and simpler designs initially – flowers, polka dots and larger wording are a good place to start. Geometric designs are great for practising repeat patterns, while the smaller, more intricate designs can be fiddly and difficult to master the first time. Practising first is always a good idea.

TOP TIP: When using the scalpel, hold it like a pen, as this allows more control over where you are cutting. Moving the template as well as the scalpel will help you get those hard-to-reach angles.

1. Draw or print out your chosen design onto card or acetate. If you would like to replicate the look of my curtains, I've included the design template in the back of the book.

2. Cut out your design – the easiest way to do it is with a craft scalpel knife. Scissors will work but can be a little tricky with more intricate designs.

3. Be careful what you are leaning on to cut out! Do not cut straight onto a tabletop or kitchen counter, as this will cause scratches … and your landlord will definitely not be happy! Use a cutting mat or thick piece of card.

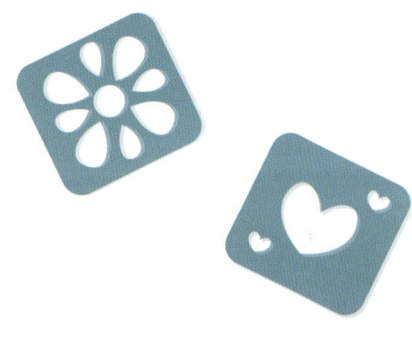

YOU WILL NEED

- ★ **Your newly made stencil**

- ★ **Curtains** – preferably a preloved pair that we can revamp and bring back to life, but if you need to buy a new pair and personalize them, that's equally as good

- ★ **Paints** – acrylics, water-based tester pots and chalk paints are ideal

- ★ **Stencil brush** or flat-headed paint brush or sponge – if using multiple colours, I would recommend a brush for each colour

- ★ **Masking tape** or **pins**

- ★ **Card** or **paper**

- ★ **Cloth**

HOW TO STENCIL CURTAINS

Grab your stencils and let's revamp those boring curtains. With a little creativity, a bit of paint and your favorite stencil you can transform your curtains into works of art that will brighten up the room and lift your mood. A super simple task, that's cost effective and so much fun. Let's go …

1. Lay your curtains out as flat as possible. If they are pretty big like mine, you might want to work on the floor.

2. Plan out your design – will you have random stencils all over the curtains? Will the design focus mainly at the bottom of the curtains like mine? Although the plan can change as you go along, it's always a good start to have something in mind.

3. Place your stencil onto the curtains and secure with masking tape.

4. Apply the paint. Dab the paint brush or sponge into the paint and then remove any excess onto a piece of

TOP TIP: It's a common mistake to add too much paint; this will cause the paint to bleed under the stencil and create blurred edges rather than sharp, crisp lines.

card or paper. We want the brush to be damp with paint, not wet. Try dabbing on a separate piece of paper before you go to your stencil to make sure you don't have too much paint.

5. Apply the paint to your stencilled area using a dabbing motion, being sure to press down the edges of the stencil as you go. Cover the entire area of the stencil with this motion. If you feel you need to add more paint, you can go over it using the same technique.

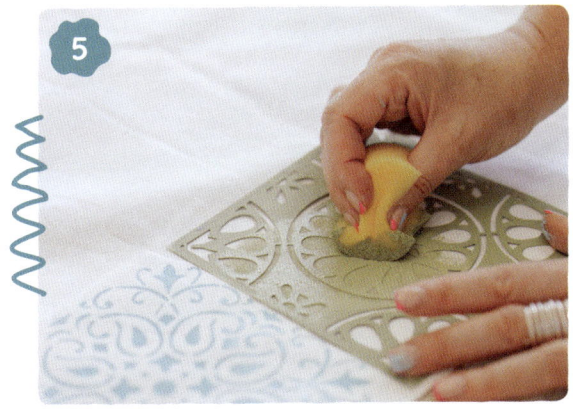

6. Remove your stencil and admire your handiwork. If you are repeating your stencil, make sure you clean the stencil before applying it to another area of your curtains. If your stencil is acetate, you can use a dry cloth. If your stencil is card, you will need to wait for the paint to dry, but as you haven't used too much paint, this shouldn't take long. Try repeating your stencil with different colours and in different directions. You could even try layering your stencils.

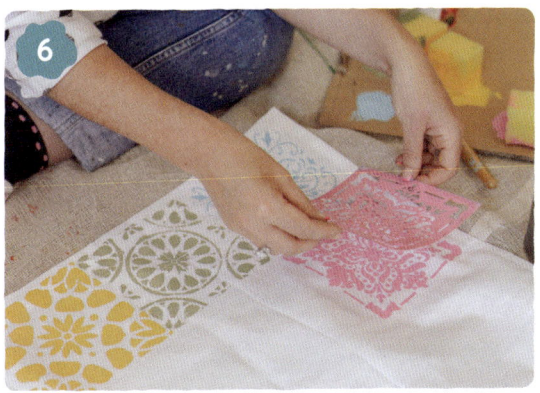

⊕ Some stunning effects can be achieved with stencils and the possibilities really are endless. You can use stencils throughout your home on walls, floors, furniture, soft furnishings or even clothing.

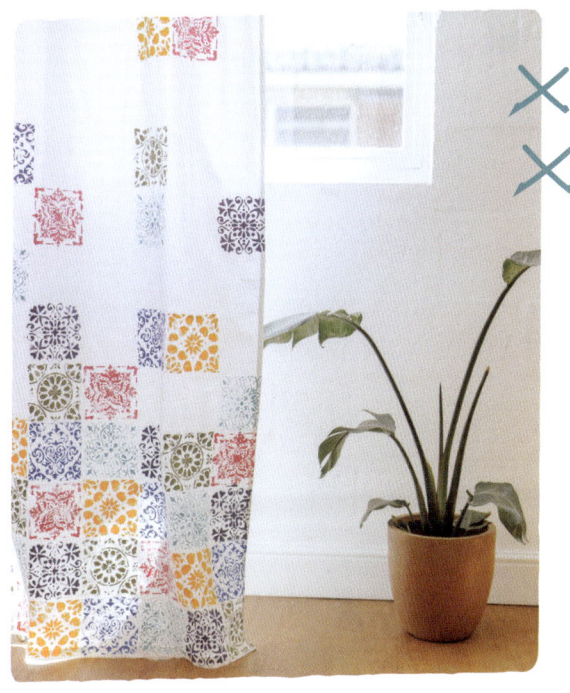

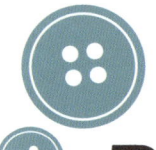

BUTTON THE BLUES

It's so important for our mental health to keep dreaming about our future, our goals, no matter how big or small. There was once a time when I didn't see a future for myself. I saw nothing ahead of me and I felt I had nothing to look forward to. When I started to make button jewellery, I felt a glimmer of hope. Maybe I did have a purpose, a reason, value …

I'm a big fan of making lists. My mum is the same. We make a list of the things we want to do, the things we want to buy and the things we would like to achieve. She often brings her list around to my house and talks me through it over coffee. Top of my list at the moment is write a book! Top of my mum's is paint the bathroom. We all need something to aim for, no matter how big or small. This is why we love booking a holiday; it gives us something to look forward to, a reason to keep going.

Loss

We all dream, we all have desires. But when we experience a loss, whether that be the death of a loved one or the end of a relationship, our dreams and hopes for the future can come crashing down. When I was severely depressed, it was the darkest time of my life. It was many years after losing Sean. I was in my early twenties, just out of university. I'd finished my studies in Bristol and moved back home to Liverpool. Studying was the thing that had kept me going. When Sean died, school and studying became my focus, my distraction. But now, it was all gone, it was done! What now? A diploma, a degree and a master's had all been achieved. But I felt no satisfaction. I didn't experience a sigh of relief or excitement at the chance of freedom that lots of people enjoy when they finish studying. For me, it was another loss. Another dramatic change to my life that I had to come to terms with.

I felt like I was returning home to sorrow, to the place where I had experienced so much pain. My friends were scattered across the country. My loneliness was overwhelming. It felt like only a matter of weeks before I spiralled back into my grief. I must admit I was desperate to end it all. Fortunately, I was too strong to do anything about it, although at the time it felt quite the opposite. I told myself I was a failure, weak, a coward. I would punch walls, pinch my skin and pull at my hair. There were days, even weeks, where I wouldn't see daylight. I hid away in my bed, the hours and days just passing me by. Time went quickly and slowly all at once. I slept and slept and slept, I was so tired, tired of who I was and tired of my life. The constant relentless emotions exhausted me.

I was single, living at home with no job. My only responsibility was walking Prince, the dog, so, I would resentfully wander the streets with Prince while I sobbed. Is this it? What's the point? Why am I here? I had no purpose and, quite frankly, I didn't want one.

Finding a purpose

One day, my grandad gave me a tin of buttons. He was creative and he knew I was too. He knew I could put them to good use. I was never one to throw anything away, even when I was younger. Among the dark days I did have ok ones. Some days were easier than others, at least. It was on one of those easier days that I picked up the tin and started making button jewellery. I threaded the buttons onto lengths of string and made necklaces and bracelets. I reluctantly enjoyed the process. Being depressed had become my normal, it was my everyday, and although painful, it was familiar. A distraction to this familiarity was unsettling.

But I was enjoying making the jewellery, and the bracelets and necklaces actually looked cool! I started to gain confidence and to feel almost proud of what I was creating. It wasn't too taxing. It was something I could do from bed or sitting in front of the TV. I didn't need expensive equipment or a huge workspace. It wasn't a messy or time-consuming activity, so I could pick it up and drop it as and when I wanted to.

It gave me a purpose; even if it was making "silly" button jewellery, it was something. Friends and family liked what I was making, and a few people even wanted to buy my jewellery. Initially I wasn't very good at it. Although the necklaces looked good, they weren't very secure – a bit like me at the time! It's just as well they were going only to family and friends, as they fell apart after a few wears. But you've got to start somewhere, right? With time and practice, I found out which materials worked best to create quality products. So let me share with you this simple technique for making button jewellery. Whether you're making button jewellery for yourself or as a gift for someone else, this activity is a great one for keeping your hands busy and your mind focused.

BUTTON JEWELLERY

- -

**Creating button jewellery is a super-simple activity that
keeps your hands occupied and your mind from overthinking.
It's great for all ages – kids love this one.**

Buttons can be expensive to buy, especially if you need a lot – and for this activity you do. But charity shops usually have tins filled with them, as they cut them off the clothing that doesn't make it to the shop floor. I visit my local charity shops regularly. A lot of them know me now and put their buttons to one side for me.

If you have clothes that you've grown out of, or clothes from a loved one, then you could use the buttons from those garments to make your jewellery extra special.

YOU WILL NEED

★ **Buttons** – lots of them for a necklace similar to the one i'm making you will need between 50 and 80 buttons, depending on size. Buttons come in a variety of shapes, sizes and colours. You can make various styles of jewellery depending on the buttons you use. Those small white shirt buttons make great necklaces that can be worn with anything.

★ Waxed cord

★ Scissors

★ **Ribbon** (optional)

★ **Jewellery fastening** (if making small necklaces or bracelets)

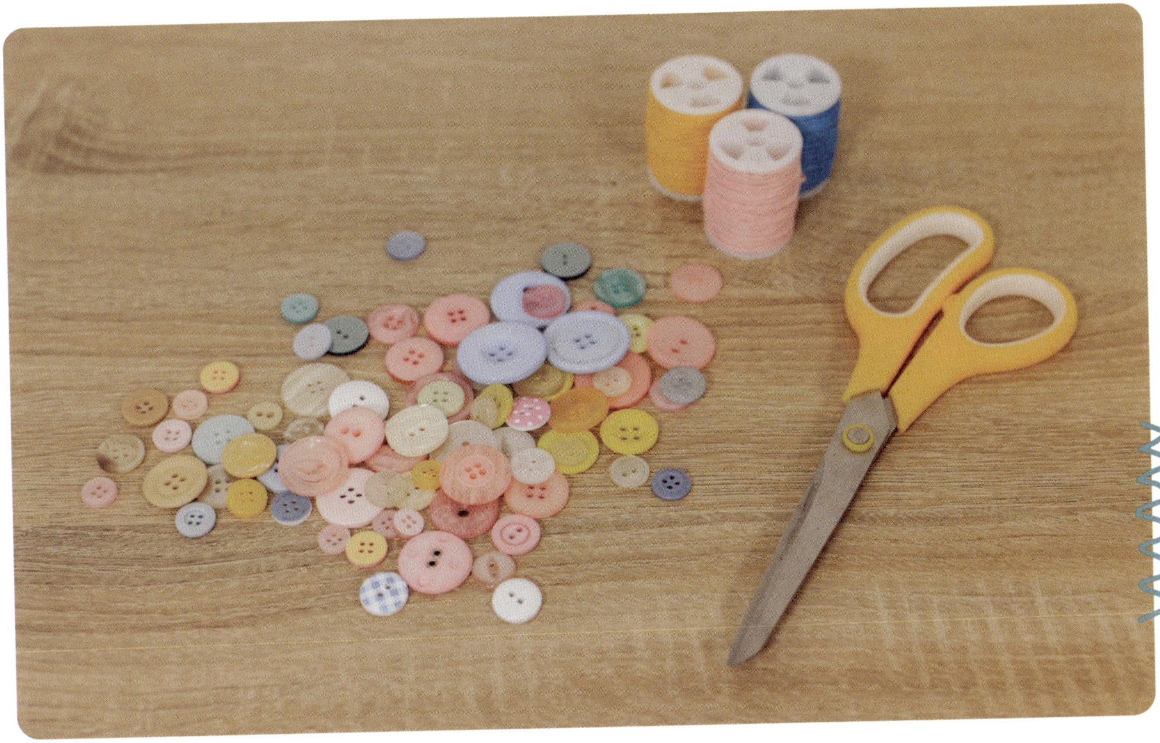

HOW TO MAKE A BUTTON NECKLACE

1. Take your waxed cord and cut it to the size you want for your piece of jewellery. I am making a long necklace that I can wear in different ways, so my cord here is 90cm/36in long. Add around 5cm/2in at the end so that you can tie a knot.

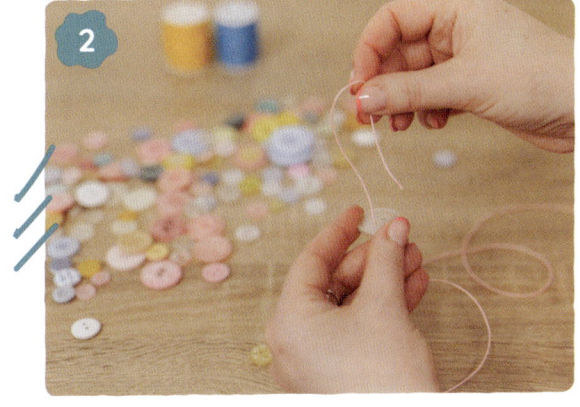

2. Thread your buttons onto the cord using the buttonholes. If the button has two holes, thread the cord through both holes.

3. If the button has four holes, still only thread the cord through two holes.

4. Keep threading until you have achieved your desired length, making sure you are pushing your buttons along the cord so they sit next to each other, leaving no gaps.

5. When you are coming to the end of your cord, leave 5cm/2in at each end and tie with a knot.

6. A sturdy knot is great for these longer necklaces, but if you are wanting to make shorter necklaces or bracelets, you will need some jewellery fastening to tie your cord to.

7. You could then tie a ribbon over the knot, for decoration.

8. Wear with pride and expect lots of lovely comments!

⊕ I like the metaphor of a button. It holds things together, a fastening that secures and opens. That's exactly what buttons did for me: they held me together. This activity helped to get me out of a very dark place. Of course, I then became a little button-obsessed and began creating all sorts of crafts with buttons – which is why when it came to naming my business years later, The Button Boutique seemed fitting!

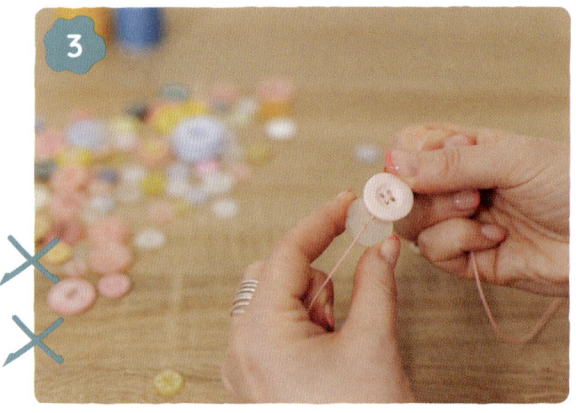

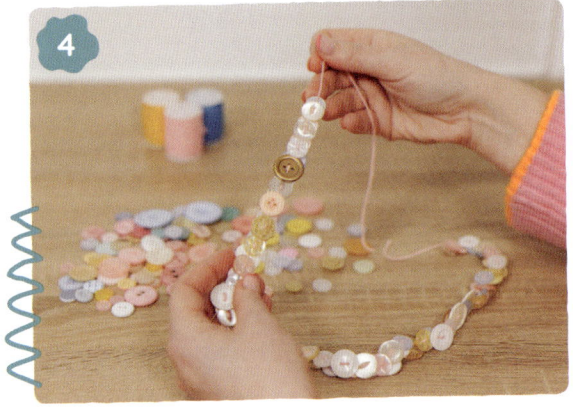

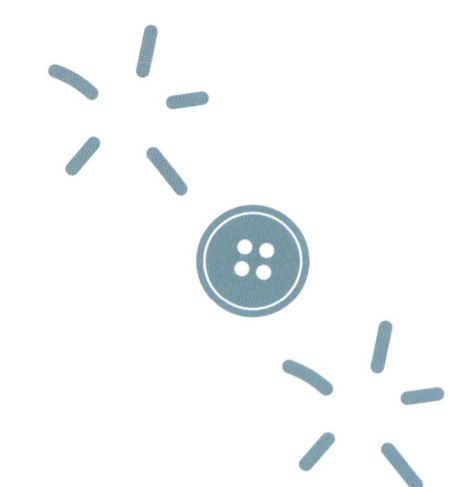

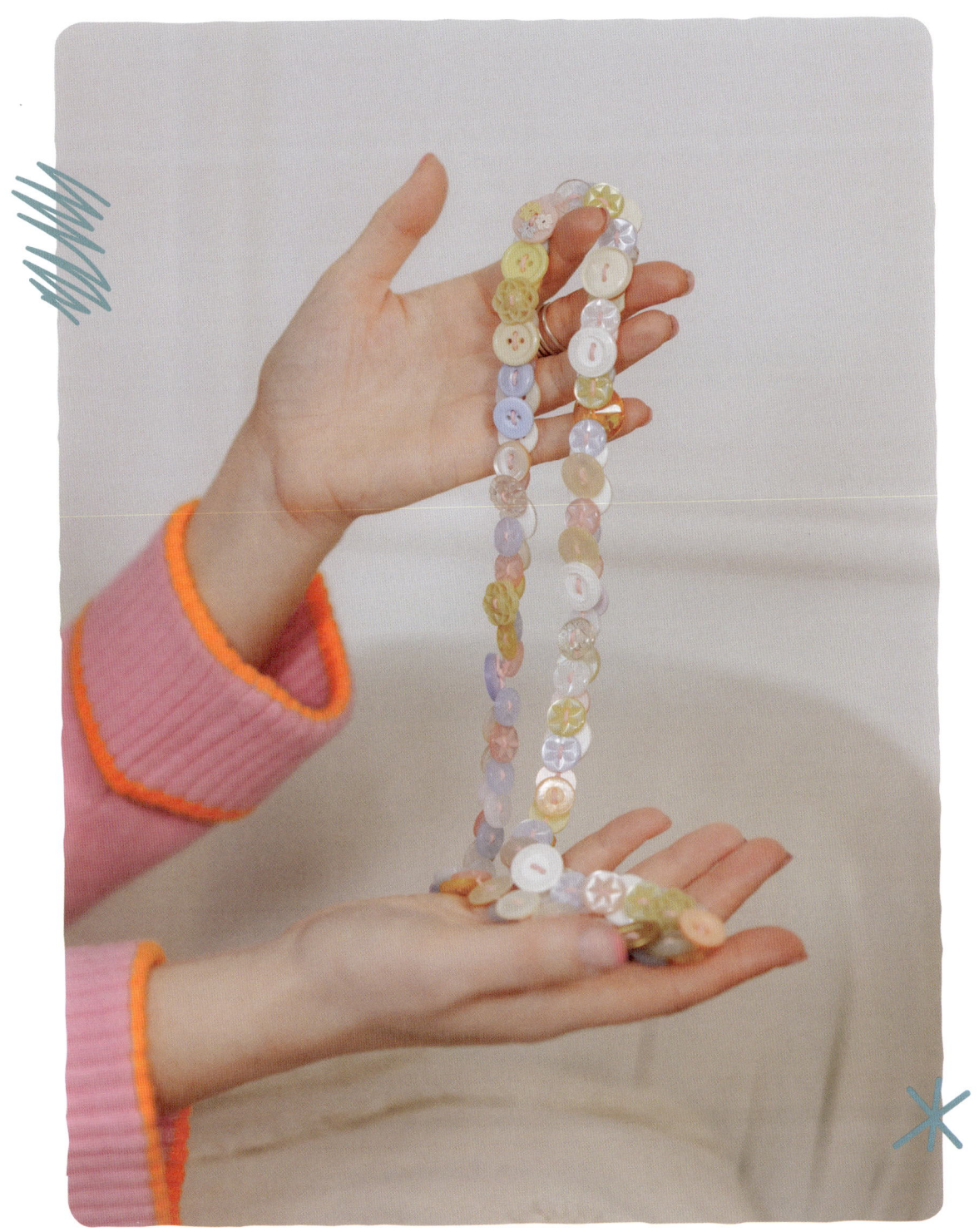

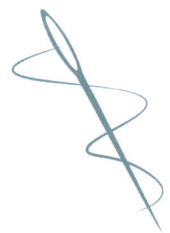
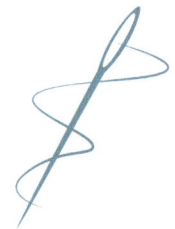

DECORATIVE MENING

Upcycling clothing allows us to be creative with our wardrobe, extends the life of preloved items, saves us money and, of course, is a sustainable option, as it prevents items from going to landfill. I see upcycling as a method for turning negatives into positives, revamping an item from redundant to reused and cherishing items of clothing that hold special memories. One way in which we can upcycle clothing is by mending them.

I'm sure you will all agree that clothes hold memories. I've talked about how Sean's clothes hold many precious memories for me: T-shirts reminding me of days out during the summer holidays, his pjs telling stories of cozy nights in front of the TV and that special red belt that he gained in his karate tournament.

Many items of my own clothes hold special memories. Looking through my wardrobe is like looking through a photograph album. If I have a particularly vivid or special memory, I can often picture exactly what I was wearing. My latest purchase was a blue tie-dye dress that I bought for my trip to Nice for my fortieth birthday. Regardless of how often I wear this dress, it will always be my Nice dress and remind me of the special days I spent

with my friends, drinking champagne at the beach bar and chatting for hours to my friend Jenny in the warm sun. I do hope this dress will stay in my wardrobe for many years to come.

Although I am a sucker for a new outfit, I do find joy in the ones I already own. When possible I will rewear and repair the classic garments I have, the garments that hold dear memories and tell special stories.

I still have my nan's scarf. When I was leaving her house to walk home on winter nights, she would wrap it around me under my coat and secure it with a huge safety pin. It was rather restricting, almost like a straitjacket, but she thought it would keep my back warm. I'm not sure why my back was so exposed! This scarf still makes an appearance every winter. Over the years it has become a little damaged but I always choose to repair it over buying a new version. This scarf means so much more to me than a new one would.

My wedding dress is probably one of my most significant items of clothing. Like most brides to be, the dress was everything and I visited lots of bridal shops and tried on many dresses in the search for "the one". I was lucky that my mum accompanied me on my dress search. We always made the day of it – a nice lunch, a glass or two of bubbles and maybe a fancy dinner afterwards. The dress search was an occasion itself.

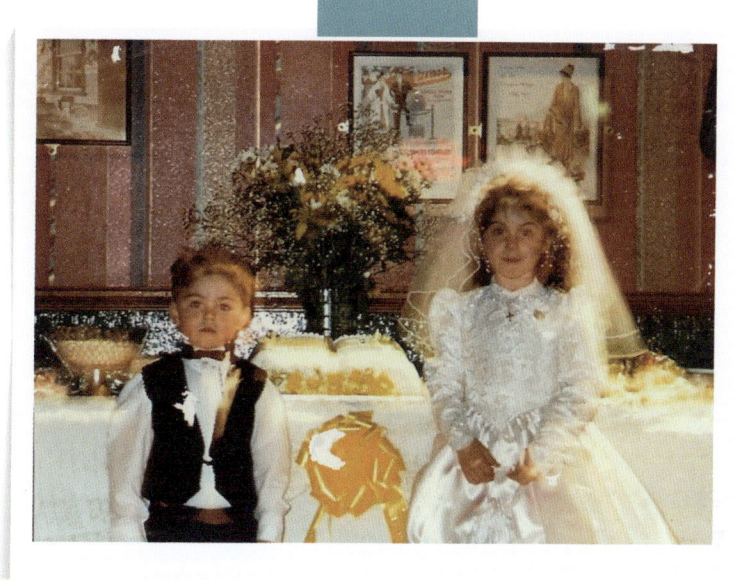

I finally found the one, a beautiful floor-length sequin gown with a lace back and covered in beads ... stunning. The dress wasn't cheap, but Mum insisted on paying for it and saved for me to have it.

I won't bore you with the details, but I didn't end up getting married on my wedding day. But to me the dress still holds special memories because it tells a story of the relationship between my mum and me. This is why I never parted with the dress – and the fact that it is a beauty. In fact, during the process of writing this book, I upcycled my wedding dress! I decided the dress needed a new dream, so I've had it altered; it now lives on as a top and skirt.

Now I see the dress as a white satin sequined version of myself – transformed from the whole experience with a lot more to give! I still have hope for my happily ever after; like the dress, it may be altered a little but is just as fabulous as the original. And I'm still a hopeless romantic who wears her heart on her sleeve. In fact, adding a heart to an item of clothing is one of my favourite ways to mend or revamp!

WEAR YOUR HEART ON YOUR SLEEVE

I must admit I'm quite a messy person who is generally surrounded by paint, so of course it ends up on my clothes. Most of the time I love it … It's a vibe! But if I want to cover a stain up, I like to add little hearts to my clothing. They look cute and are great for mending tears too. The hearts show that my items are mended with love, they mean something to me and they hold a little story.

If you spot a little heart on an item I'm wearing, know that it's probably been in my possession for a while and can certainly tell a tale or two.

However, my hearts are not reserved for my most cherished garments; they can be necessary on more recent purchases too. I recently bought a jumper, a simple grey sweatshirt, comfy and casual. Within 10 minutes, it had paint on the sleeve. As I already have several painting jumpers, I'm going to mend this one as one of my few paint-free options. Now and again it's nice to wear something that doesn't have paint on it!

YOU WILL NEED

★ **An item of clothing** – one that is torn, damaged, stained or just in need of a revamp – I've got my new grey jumper with its paint stain

★ **Contrasting fabric for the heart/s** – this could be bought fabric or another item of clothing destined for the bin. I'm using a tea towel that I just love the colour of (pink!)

★ **Thread** – embroidery threads are better for this as they are thinner and will give a more prominent stitch

★ **Sewing needle**

★ **Sharp pointed scissors**

★ **Pins** or an **embroidery hoop**

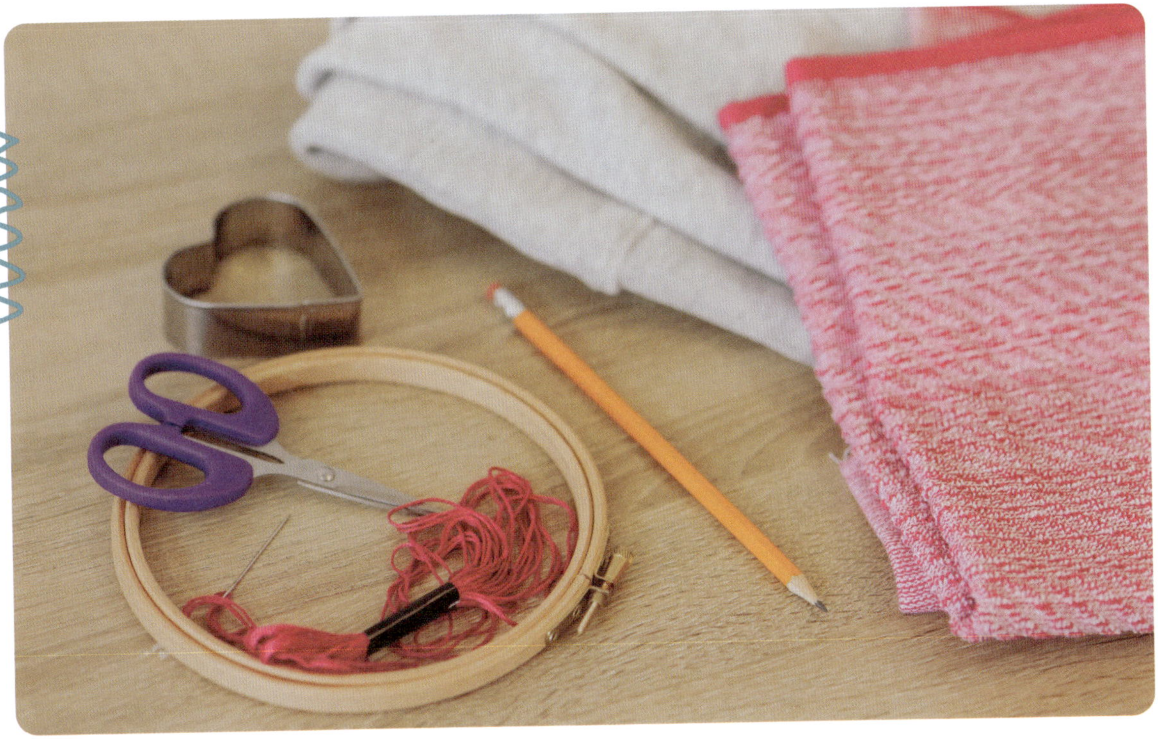

HOW TO WEAR YOUR HEART ON YOUR SLEEVE

1. Locate your stain. Mine is on the sleeve. There's often paint all over my sleeves.

2. Draw a heart onto your clothing item to cover your stain or marking. If you have something heart-shaped to hand like my cookie cutter then use this. I've included a heart template at the back of the book for you to cut out and draw around.

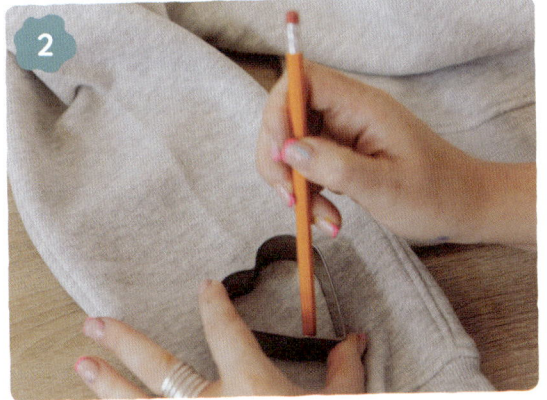

3. Place your contrasting fabric under the heart – so the inside of the sleeve in this case – and use an embroidery hoop or pin it in place. This can be a little fiddly if like me you are working a sleeve.

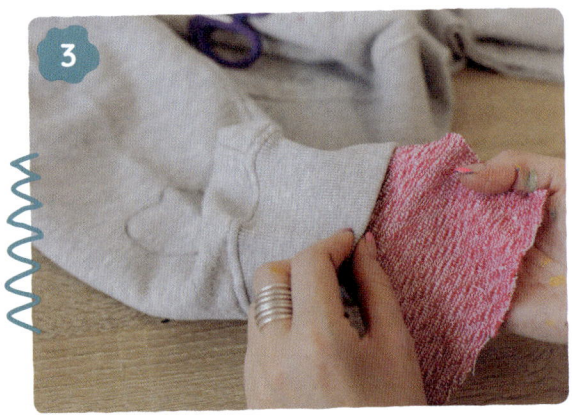

4. Thread your needle and, using a basic line stitch, stitch around the heart you have marked on the outside of the sleeve. (You are stitching both the jumper and the contrasting fabrics together.) Secure your stitches by tying a knot in your thread.

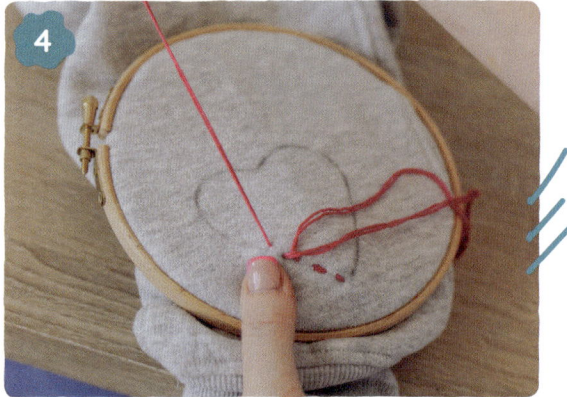

5. Using sharp pointed scissors, cut away the heart shape out of the jumper to reveal the contrasting fabric underneath. Make sure you cut within the stitched outline.

6. Trim any excess fabric from inside the sleeve.

⊕ Your heart is now on your sleeve for everyone to see. We no longer need to hide our emotions, let's wear them with pride.

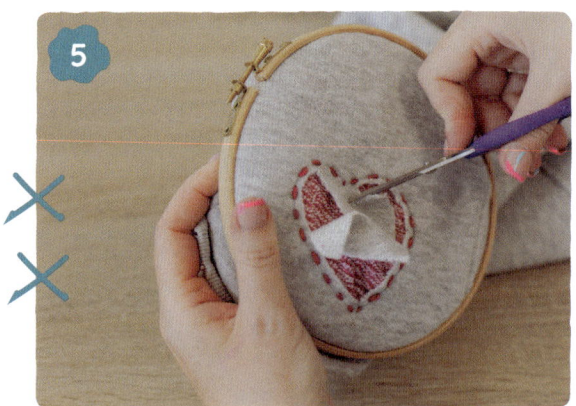

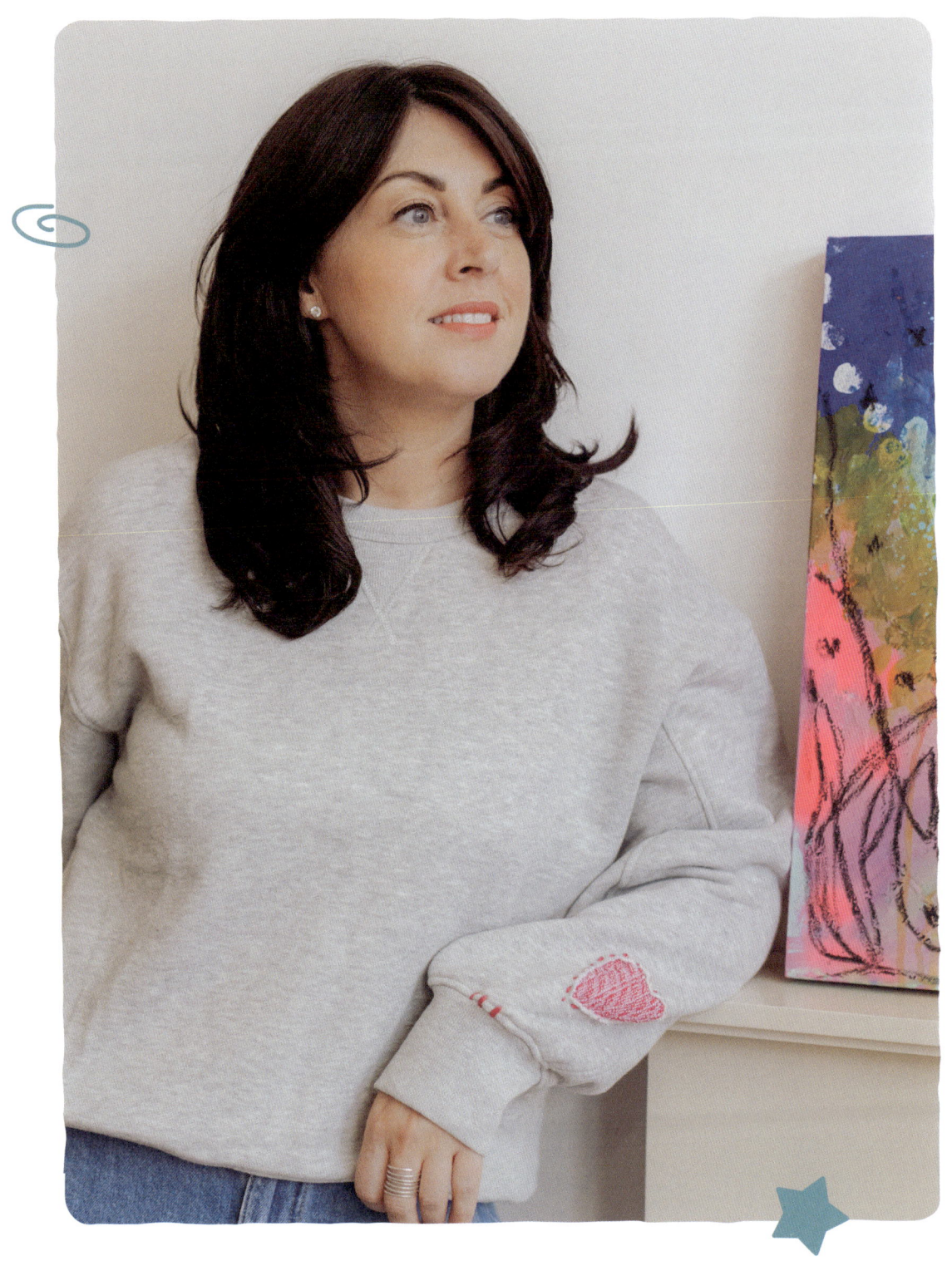

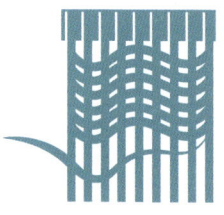

WEAVING WONDERS

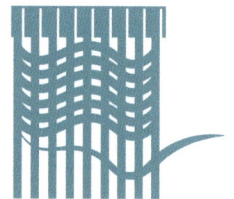

I've always had my wardrobe go-tos, the items I feel comfortable in. So when they become stained or torn, I will do my best to mend them. Repairing, upcycling and customizing our clothing is a great way to show our creativity and create one-of-a-kind items that express our personality and style – and a great way to do this is with weaving.

The history of mending clothes is a rich tapestry that reflects our resourcefulness as humans. It shows our evolving cultural attitudes toward clothing and sustainability. Mending clothes has evolved from a skill for survival to a deliberate act of creativity.

Fabric weaving is more commonly used for repairing torn clothing, a technique where new threads are interwoven into the damaged area of a garment to restore its original appearance. This method is often used to repair small holes, tears, or worn-out areas. When done well, fabric weaving repairs are nearly invisible, maintaining the garment's original appearance.

However, you can also use this method to create custom patches in your clothing, using contrasting colours and fabrics to add colour, texture and some serious style.

My painting jeans

My painting jeans represent so much; they are a key item in my wardrobe. They symbolize all that I love about myself, my creativity, my passions, my energy.

I see them as a work of art. I wear my painting jeans a lot, for all my workshops, classes, one-to-one sessions and my own creative projects. They've visited hospitals, festivals, hotels and parties. They hold a variety of paints from a variety of projects ... I can see the grey paint from the hotel refurbishment, the yellow from the Italian restaurant table and the pink from my living room walls.

My painting jeans remind me of who I am, what I've done and what I'm aiming for. They are messy and colourful, which is pretty much me in a nutshell.

My painting jeans go through a lot, they get a good deal of use and often tear at the knees. I frequently have to repair them, but if anything, this often adds character to them and makes them more valuable to me.

Dopamine dressing

You've heard me say it before, and I'm going to say it again: I love bright colours and I love to wear them as often as possible. When I'm not in my painting jeans, I wear colourful outfits, and it lifts my mood and puts a smile on the faces of those around me.

These days, I tend to do a bit of networking, getting myself out there and telling my story to anyone who will listen, and I always wear bright or bold colours when I do. I've found it gets me noticed – even in a crowded room, you won't lose sight of me!

"Dopamine dressing" is on the up and it's become a huge trend on social media. If you don't know what dopamine dressing is, it is the concept of wearing clothes that boost your mood and increase happiness. It involves choosing outfits based on colours, styles and textures that evoke positive emotions and enhance your overall wellbeing.

I have a Barbie-pink jacket that never fails to lift my mood; pink is one of my favourite colours, so it always makes me smile. The jacket even has shoulder pads, which makes me appear confident even if I don't feel it. Usually within a hour of wearing it, I start to feel my confidence grow! So on the days when I need to be at my best, my pink jacket is my go-to.

And then I have my rainbow trainers which are covered in coloured stones. Whenever I wear them, they make me want to dance. I find myself walking a little more elegantly, pointing my toes with each step in the hope that a passerby will notice them. I love it when I get compliments on them; they are fabulous, so the compliments come thick and fast.

I actually wore both my pink jacket and rainbow trainers for the photoshoot for this book and I was on fire that day! Should anything ever happen to either of these power pieces, I will have to get my sewing needle out immediately to repair them!

I'm always looking for fun and unique ways to add colour to my wardrobe and make me stand out from the crowd. The heart patches on pages 106–8 are a great way to do this, but another way to revamp your clothes is with decorative weaving.

DECORATIVE WEAVING

This decorative weaving activity celebrates the imperfections and makes a feature of them, as well as adding colour to your preloved clothes. This is a fun and resourceful way to make one-of-a-kind items!

Decorative weaving is a simple but effective technique that is a great one for saving clothes and saving time. It's pretty easy to do and does not take hours of stitching, adding colour and personality to clothing in a matter of minutes. It's great for most items of clothing but particularly effective on harder-wearing items such as jeans and jackets.

I have a pair of jeans that have paint on and a tear in the leg. I wear them a lot! I'm going to repair them by adding a little colour and enhancing the tear rather than disguising it. As you will be aware by now, I'm a big fan of pink, so I will add some pink threads and fabrics so I can wear these jeans with my other clothes ... I'm thinking of my pink power jacket!

YOU WILL NEED

★ **A torn item of clothing** – to repair. You could also customize new items with this mending activity

★ **Colourful/patterned fabrics** – these could be fabrics from old clothes, or new, unused fabrics

★ **Wool, ribbons** and **laces** – optional, but great for adding colour and texture

★ **Sewing needle** and **scissors**

★ **Thread**

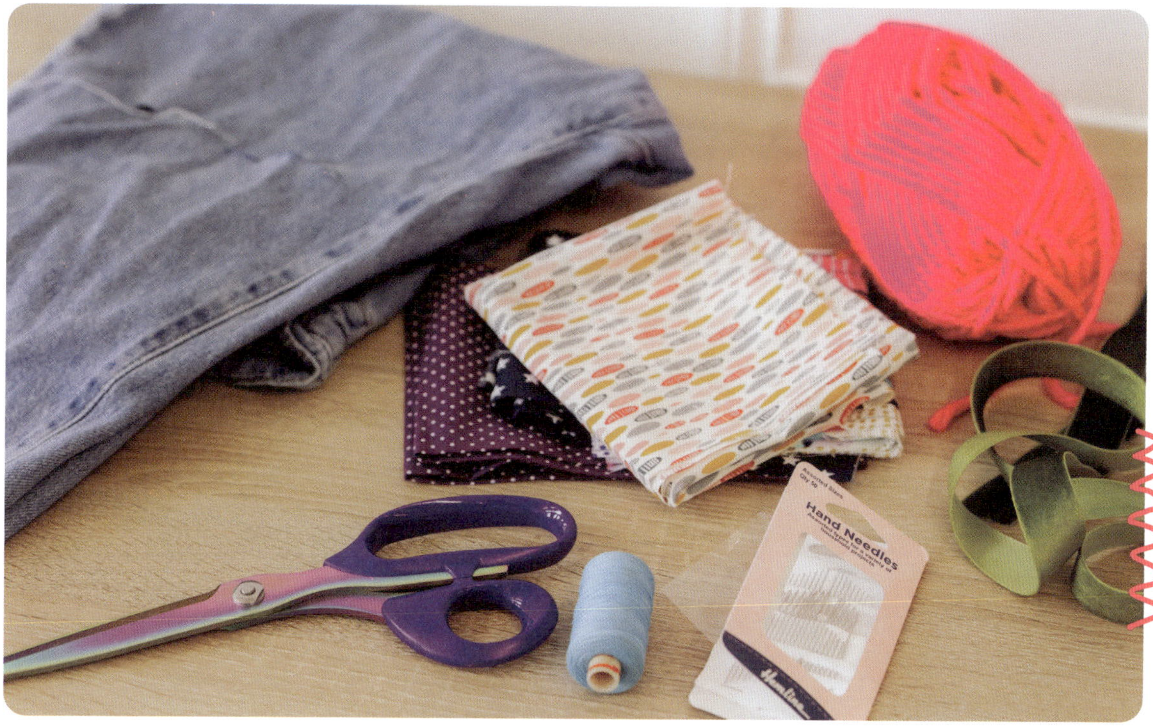

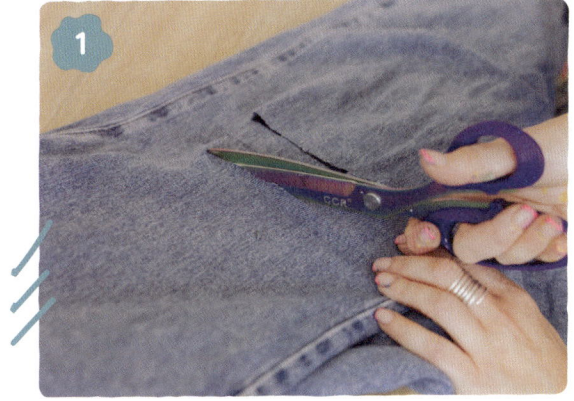

HOW TO MEND WITH DECORATIVE WEAVING

1. To create your weaving design you will need more than one tear. So depending on your item of clothing, you may need to add tears or widen/enlarge a tear using scissors. Use your scissors to create tears that sit next to each other. I had one original tear in my jeans. I'm adding two more tears approx 15cm/6in in length to give me a larger surface for my weaving design.

2. Cut or tear your colourful/patterned fabrics into 2.5cm/1in strips. Make sure the strips are long enough to weave through the tears.

3. Weave the fabric strips in and out of the tears.

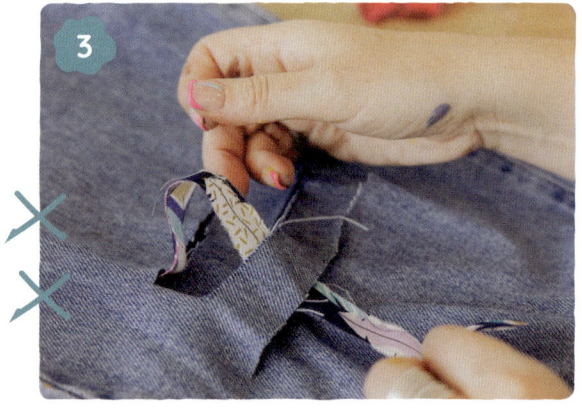

4. Secure the strips by stitching in place at the top and bottom, a simple tacking stitch will hold the fabric in place and you will need to secure each time by knotting at the back.

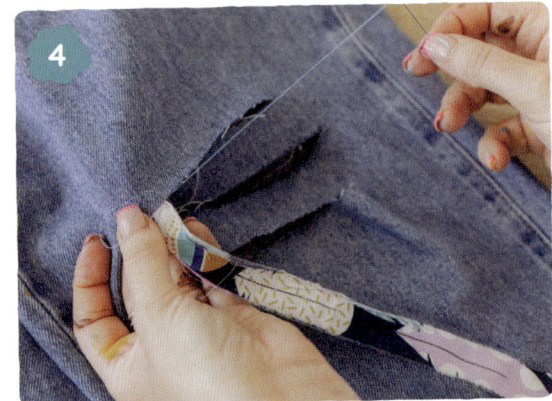

5. You can do the same with wool, ribbons and laces to add texture and colour to your woven design.

6. And that's it – it's super simple but a very effective way of adding colour to your clothing. Wear the items with pride and feel your confidence grow.

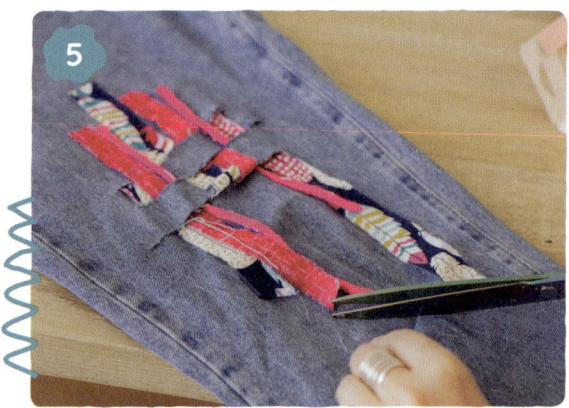

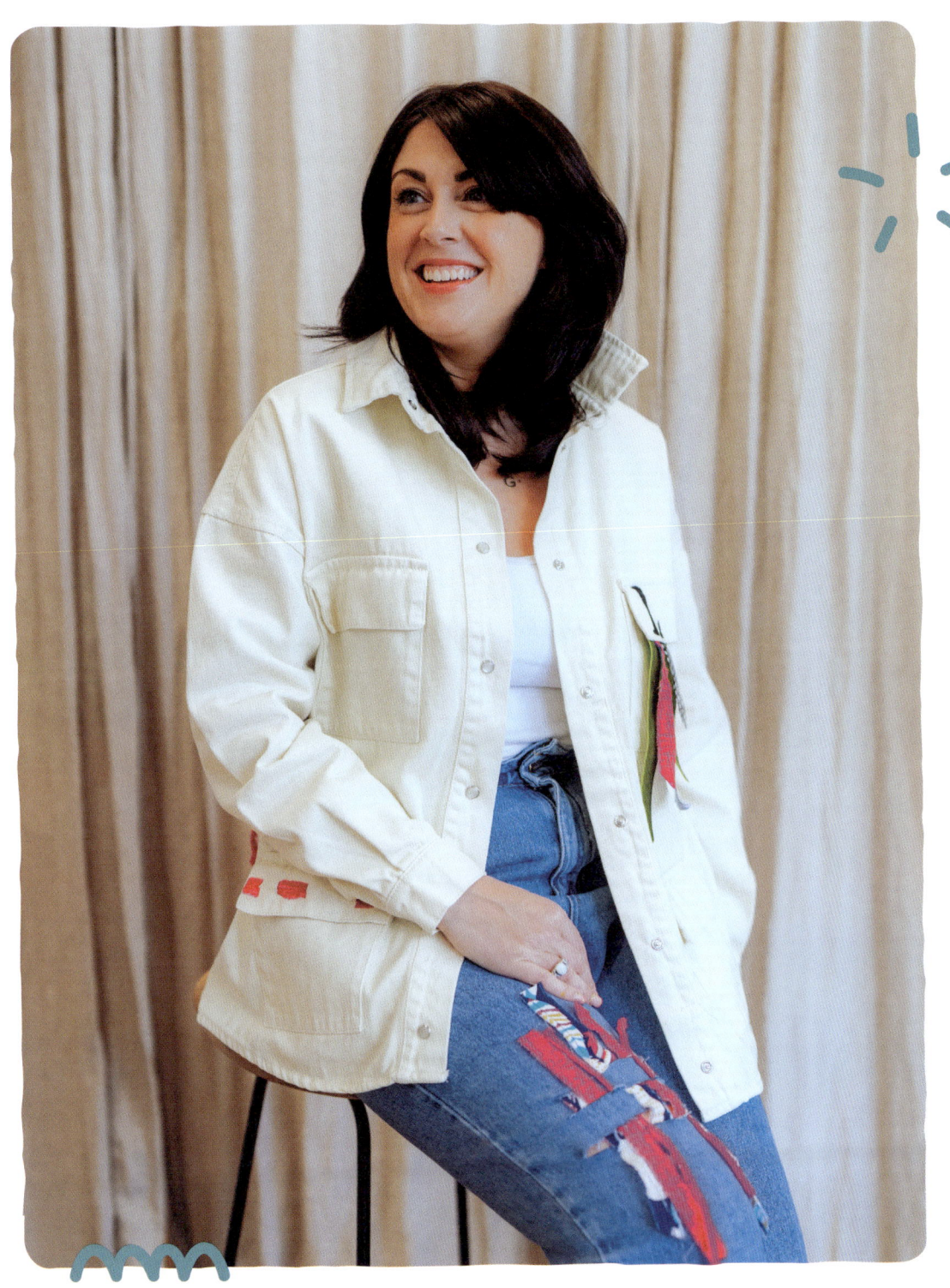

 # DECOUPAGE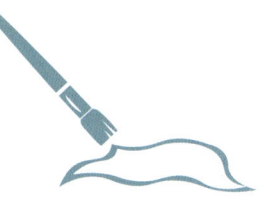

In a nutshell, decoupage is a crafting technique that involves decorating surfaces with paper and glue. Decoupage is one of my favourite crafts, as it's super easy and so much fun. You don't need expensive materials or to be an expert crafter to produce something beautiful and unique.

When I'm working with the little ones, I describe this technique to them as cutting and sticking, to which they reply:

I can do that!

And I reply:

Yes, you can.

And so can you!

Decoupage is a great mindfulness activity, as you can completely switch off while you do it. Much like other repetitive crafts, such as knitting and sewing, you don't have to overthink it. Once you're in your rhythm, your hands take over and you just create. I find it similar to meditation. It has been proven that entering this state is beneficial to our mental health, relieving stress, anxiety and depression. Additionally, taking time for mindfulness activities, such as

decoupage, can lower our blood pressure and give us a better quality of sleep.

The word "decoupage" originates from the French word *découper*, which means to cut out or to cut from something. It's a great art form for using up scrap papers such as newspapers, magazines, tissue paper, wrapping paper and even photographs. It's also a perfect craft for making with paper keepsakes – those little paper memories that can be so sentimental or nostalgic, but you just don't know what to do with them.

Decoupage is also a great activity for all ages and is an ideal project for teaching reusing and recycling to children. It shows the transformation that happens when you take something unused and repurpose it into something special and meaningful. Sustainable box, ticked!

Pretty much anything can be decoupaged. I love to decoupage

furniture, as it is a great way of adding colour, texture and detail to simple items quickly and affordably (see pages 162–5). Picture frames, trays, boxes, vases and jam jars also make great projects. It's a versatile and accessible crafting technique that allows for endless creativity and personalization. With a little practice and experimentation, you can create beautiful and unique decoupage pieces to enhance your home, or to give as gifts. My mum has many picture frames I've decorated on display with photos of myself and Sean.

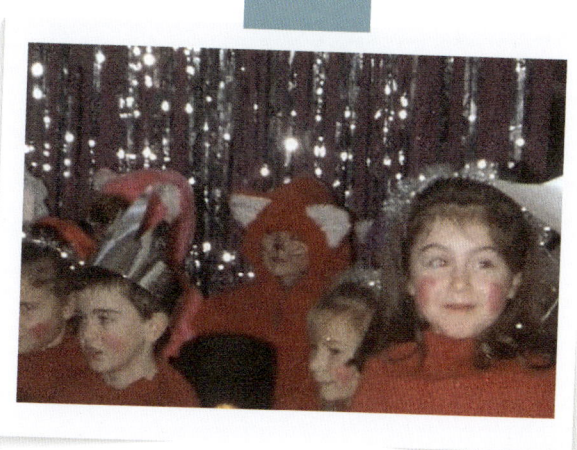

Bus tickets

Sean liked to collect things. His collections chopped and changed regularly. They never really grew all that large, but he used to put all his findings in his "private drawer", which was strictly out of bounds to my mum and me.

Whenever we would get the bus into town, he would keep hold of the bus tickets. I remember one day Sean asked the bus driver if he had any spare tickets to add to his collection. He was delighted when the driver gave him an entire roll of tickets that had never been used. These went into his private drawer, never to be seen again!

When he died, we did gain access to the private drawer and found lots of silly little things, like a small collection of can ring pulls, a bag of marbles, some pinecones and key rings. His spy file was also in there, which he'd got from Book Day at school – a day when the school asked parents to give their kids money to buy a book. I'm sure my mum couldn't afford to give us that money, but we never went without. So, Sean got his spy file, even if it was the last thing he needed at that point. Nevertheless, that spy file has become a treasured item for both my mum and me, so I suppose it was worth eating beans on toast for.

Anyway, back to the bus tickets. I wish I had those bus tickets today. I would love to decoupage a picture frame with them and display a photograph of us all during one of our trips into town. What a wonderful project that would make. I don't have the tickets, but I do have a frame, so let's get decoupaging.

DECOUPAGE PICTURE FRAME

I have many photographs of myself and my brother when we were children. They are not stored on a phone for me to look back on whenever I want to. I don't want these photos to sit in a drawer for nobody to see, so I display them with pride.

I love picture frames and have so many of them around my house with photos, drawings and even sentimental keepsakes inside. Often a frame can really enhance an image, so it's wonderful when the frame itself can become part of the sentiment of what's displayed inside.

I'm going to decoupage a frame that brings myself and my brother together. I'll use papers with patterns and words that remind me of him, the love that we shared, as well as many of my favourite colours, so it fits well in my home.

YOU WILL NEED

★ **Frame** – you may have old frames around the house, but if not, take yourself to your local charity shop and have a good rummage. Charity shops are great for affordable one-of-a-kind items for craft projects. I've chosen a wide frame, as there is more surface area to decoupage.

★ **Paper** – you can buy decoupage paper, although scrap papers, tissue paper, napkins and newspapers will work just as well. Thinner paper sticks better, so avoid using thick wallpaper or card on smaller projects, such as a frame. It's a good idea to photocopy any photographs onto copy paper. Try to use papers with interesting patterns, texts and colours, as these make for beautiful projects.

If, like me, you are decoupaging in memory of someone, writing a letter to decoupage with is also a nice idea. Take a moment to write a few words to your loved one.

★ **Scissors** and/or **craft knife** (if you'll be cutting paper)

- ★ **Decoupage medium** – you can get a specific decoupage glue made for decoupage projects, but if you don't have this, PVA glue works just as well

- ★ **Brush** – use a soft bristle brush to apply the glue, as tougher bristles can tear the paper. Foam brushes and flat-head brushes work particularly well.

- ★ **Sandpaper** - depending on your frame

- ★ **Clear varnish** (optional) – can give the finished piece a glossy or matt finish, depending on the type of varnish you choose

- ★ **Embellishments** – you might want to add ribbons, buttons or sequins

HOW TO DECOUPAGE

1. Before you start, take out the glass and the back of the frame, and put this to one side until the decoupaging is finished.

2. Prepare the frame by wiping it clean and lightly sanding away any grit or

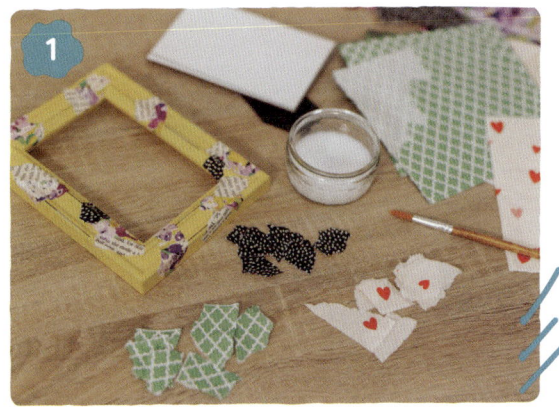

stubborn dust. You're aiming to have a smooth and clean base.

3. Tear or cut out papers and designs. This is your opportunity to be playful, to experiment and to mix up different patterns and papers. Smaller pieces of paper work better for smaller projects, such as frames. Cutting them to approximately 2.5cm x 2.5cm/ 1in x 1in is ideal.

TIP: This craft is not too messy, but it's always useful to have a damp cloth to hand for sticky fingers and any spillages. Avoid using a paper table cover for decoupage, as everything will end up stuck to the table. Believe me, it's very annoying!

4. Next, prepare your design and layout. I like to arrange my cut-outs onto my frame to make sure I'm happy with my design. You can overlap the cut-outs, layer them, or arrange them in a pattern, depending on the look you want to achieve.

5. Once you're happy with the design, it's time to start sticking. Using your brush, apply the glue evenly to the frame. If you have a large frame, work on one area at a time so your glue doesn't start to dry while you work. Apply your paper over the glue and, once in place, apply a light covering of glue over the top.

6. Repeat the process, adding glue both under and over the paper until your frame is filled.

7. Allow your frame to dry. This could take up to 6 hours, depending on how much glue you've used and the temperature of the room. The glue will dry clear. Thicker papers will start to peel off as they dry. Keep an eye on them, smoothing them out as needed.

8. Once the frame is completely dry, you can add a varnish. This isn't always necessary, but it will prevent the papers from peeling over time. It's also a good idea if you are gifting your frame, as it makes it more durable. After the glue and varnish

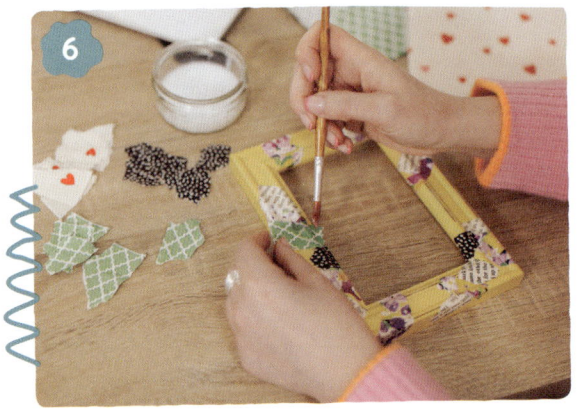

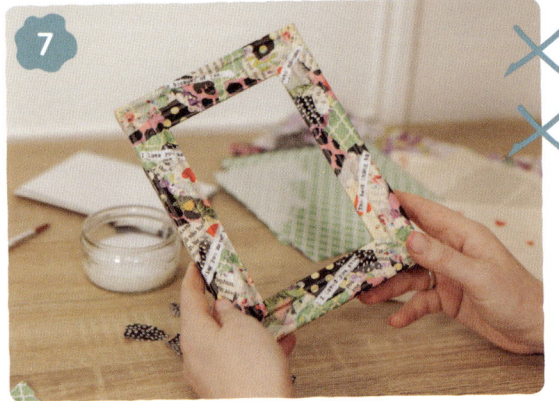

has dried completely, you can add decorative elements to enhance your decoupage project. This could include painting, stencilling, stamping or adding embellishments such as beads, sequins or ribbons.

9. Display your favourite picture in your beautiful new frame.

Now that you've decoupaged a frame, maybe you could try some other items: jam jars, wine bottles and candlestick holders are all small projects that are great for beginners.

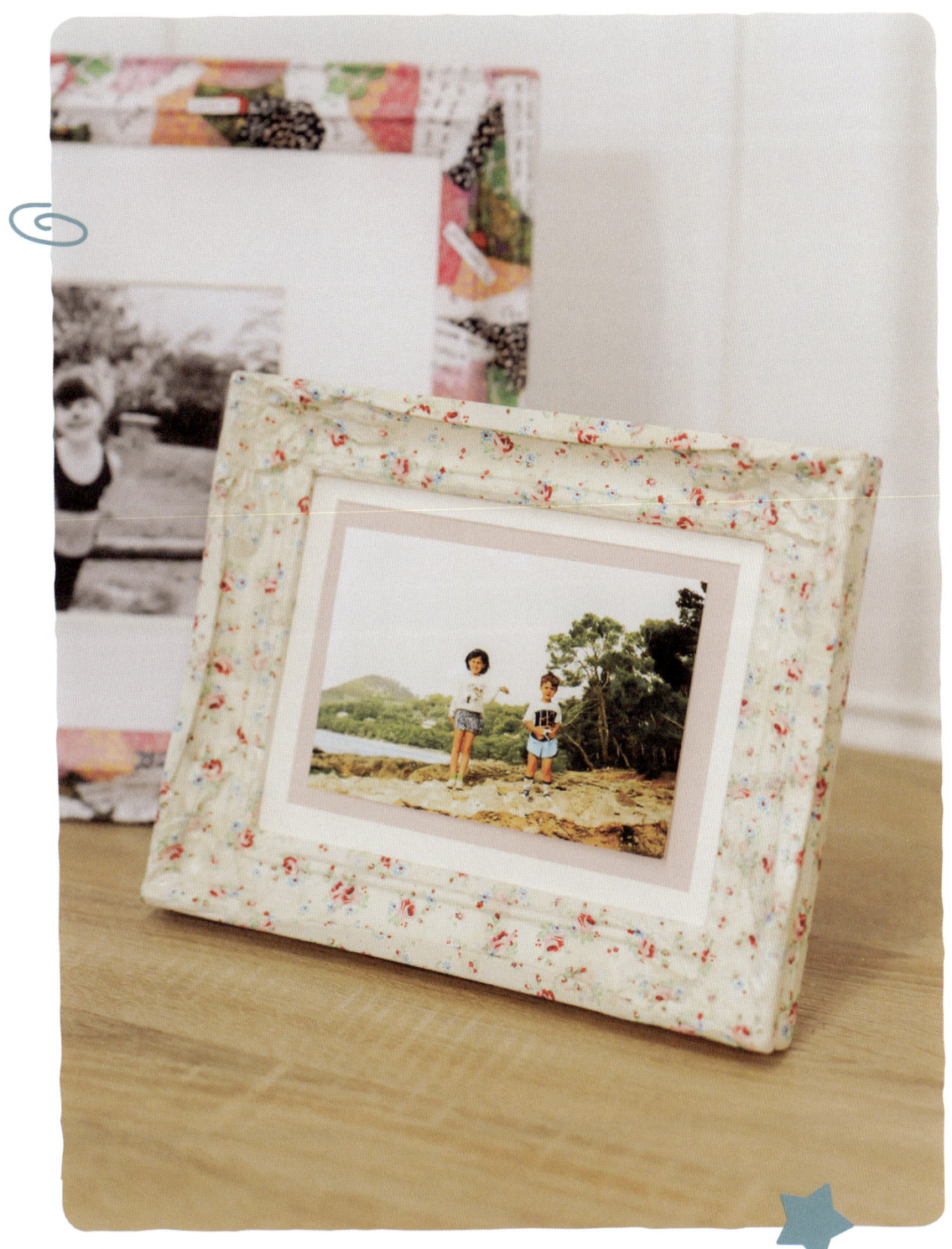

MENDING

YOUR

MIND

Mending requires care, time, patience and skill. I like to think of mending and upcycling as the transformation of turning negatives into positives through creativity.

Mending in crafting and mending your mind share profound similarities in both the process and outcome. Both involve recognizing areas that are in need of repair – whether that's a tear in fabric or a source of psychological pain – and addressing them with care and patience. Both require attention to detail and the use of techniques that restore and enhance the original.

Through my creative practice I've been able to mend my mind and lift my mood. For many years my love of upcycling has grown into a passion. It's now part of my daily life and, of course, my career. Upcycling furniture in particular has been great for my mental health. Finishing a sometimes lengthy project gives me a real sense of accomplishment, and to hear people say they love what I've done does wonders for my self-esteem and self-worth..

Mending your mind through mindfulness and self-care practices such as art and craft can be deeply personal and transformative and will lead to renewed strength and resilience. In this section, I've included some projects that allow you to see with your own eyes the transformational nature of upcycling. Through crafting, patience and skill, you can give broken, tired and old items a new lease of life – and give yourself a new lease of life too!

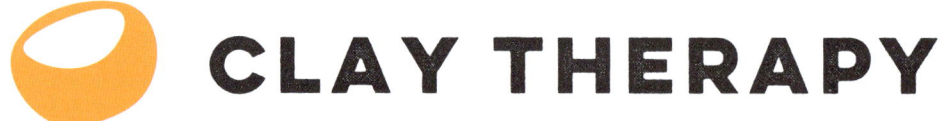# CLAY THERAPY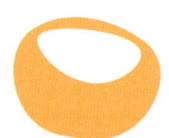

Clay therapy is a form of psychotherapy, where feelings and emotions become visible through the manipulation of the clay. It can be an alternative to talking therapy when we find it difficult to articulate our thoughts. Working with clay is a great mindfulness technique because its tactile nature encourages us to truly be in the moment.

Do you have a trigger? Something that can change your mood instantly? One minute you're happily getting on with your day, then the next minute you hear, see or smell something that brings a whole load of emotions flooding your way. These could be fond memories of your wedding day from smelling the same perfume you wore, or sadness from hearing the song that was played at your nan's funeral, or anxiety from driving past your old school.

I can't hear a Michael Jackson song without thinking of my brother, and every time I eat a jelly baby I remember my nan.

My nemesis

However, my biggest trigger is driving. Even the thought of driving makes me feel ill! Sean was hit by a car and died on impact, so for me a car is a deadly weapon. I have fought to overcome this fear since he died, but it is definitely an ongoing struggle for me.

I recently passed my driving test. It was about time – I had been taking lessons on and off for almost 20 years! Understandably, after losing Sean the way we did, driving did not come easily to me. I couldn't seem to move past the fact that this was a vehicle that killed my little brother. The anxiety I got before each lesson was horrendous, which is why it took me so long. I would take lessons, work myself up into a frenzy, then give up, telling myself driving wasn't worth it. Then a year later I would start to build up the courage to try again. It got to a point where it was no longer about the driving but more about the fact that this was something I clearly needed to overcome.

After four attempts, I passed my driving test! I was delighted, over the moon that I'd conquered my fear …

Had I heck! If anything, it got worse after passing my test because I was then faced with driving a car alone, the security of the instructor now removed. My problems had only just begun. It has been over a year and the car still sits outside the house. My nemesis. The very thought of having to drive that car can transform me from chilled to hysterical in moments.

I have forced myself to drive the car, but we are talking five occasions in total. The night before, I didn't sleep, I couldn't eat, I had a red rash all over my neck and chest. Then when I was in the car, my hands were sweaty, my legs shook and my mouth was dry.

Every day I walk past the car parked outside my house to the train station. But then I feel guilty that the car that I worked so hard to drive is sitting unused because I'm too afraid. Then I think to myself, *Is it really that big a deal if you don't drive the car? But if you don't drive the car, then what are you paying for?* It's an internal conversation I've had with myself daily since I passed my test.

Trying something new

One day, after driving to work (one of the very few occasions that happened) I arrived in a state of panic, and a colleague who was also a counsellor and therapist picked up on my distress and offered me clay therapy sessions. I wasn't sure, but I thought, *It's got to be worth a try.*

Now, even for a creative person such as myself, clay therapy was a little alien at first. I entered the session thinking I would be making bowls and vases while chatting through my feelings. Actually, it wasn't like that at all; in fact, there was not a lot of talking. It was all about allowing my emotions and energy to mould the clay. I did a quick meditation exercise with the therapist, then closed my eyes and placed my hands into the clay in front of me. It's very much a sensory experience and not being able to see what I was creating was a unique feeling for me.

I took a course of clay therapy and although it didn't help me overcome my fear of driving – I think driving will always be an issue for me – it most definitely calmed me and reduced my anxiety generally. After each session I felt relaxed and more positive.

What I found truly beneficial was the sensory element. The clay has a unique tactile quality that I found soothing. Working with clay engaged my senses more than other mediums, which I found to be extremely relaxing and strangely grounding, despite the fact that I'm a visual person and therefore I like to see what I am creating. This, combined with the mindfulness of creating something with my hands, made it an excellent activity for keeping me calm. With this in mind, I decided to go along to a few local clay workshops. The first one I went to was about pinch pots.

PINCH POTS

Pinch pots are a simple and fun activity for a clay novice such as myself. Kids will love these!

The pots are made by pinching and shaping the clay with your fingers, one of the earliest methods of pottery-making that has been used by cultures around the world for thousands of years.

I'm using air-drying clay for my pot, so it will be for decorative purposes only. Adding a varnish or lacquer at the end will make it more durable but not suitable for holding liquids.

YOU WILL NEED

★ **Clay** – air-drying clay doesn't require a kiln. For a small pot you will need a tennius ball size piece of clay

★ **A glass board, plastic mat** or **tablecloth**

★ **Water**

★ **A knife** or **scissors**

★ **Tools for printing** – such as a fork, bubble wrap or wire (optional)

★ **Paint**

★ **Paint brushes**

★ **Clear varnish** or **lacquer** (optional)

HOW TO MAKE A PINCH POT

1. Prepare your area. Clay can be messy so make sure you protect your work area with a board, mat or tablecloth and wear clothes you don't mind getting dirty – although clay, will wash off most surfaces.

2. Prepare your clay: start with a lump of clay that is soft and pliable. If your clay is too dry, you can moisten it slightly with water to make it more workable.

3. Begin by forming the base of your pinch pot. Roll the clay into a ball between your hands, then use your thumb to press into the centre of the ball, creating a hollow indentation.

4. Continue pressing and pinching the clay with your fingers to gradually widen and shape the base of the pot.

5. Create the walls – once you have formed a base, begin pinching and pulling the clay upward to form the walls of your pot. Use your thumb and fingers to gently pinch and shape the clay, rotating the pot to ensure even thickness and smoothness.

6. As you continue to pinch and shape the clay, thin out the walls of the pot to your desired thickness. Use your fingers to smooth and refine the surface of the pot, removing any lumps or imperfections. You may wish to tidy the edges with a knife or scissors.

7. Shape and decorate: experiment with different shapes and forms as you pinch and shape the clay. You can create round pots, oval pots, asymmetrical pots, or any other shape you desire. You can also add texture or decoration to the surface of the pot by pressing objects into the clay or carving designs with a tool, for example a fork.

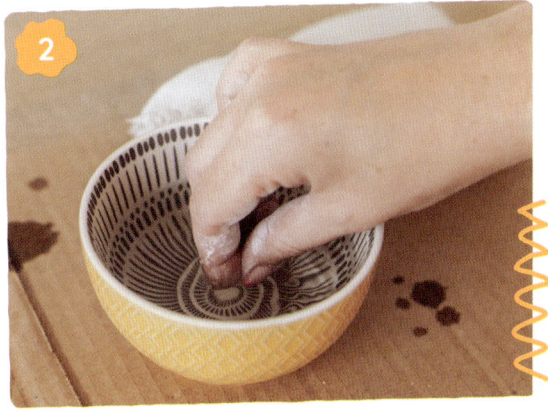

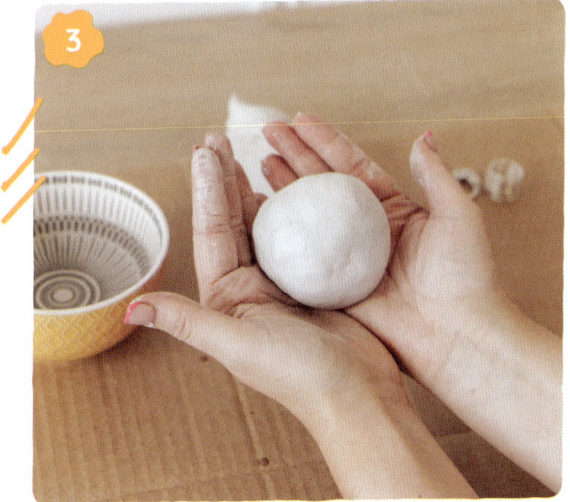

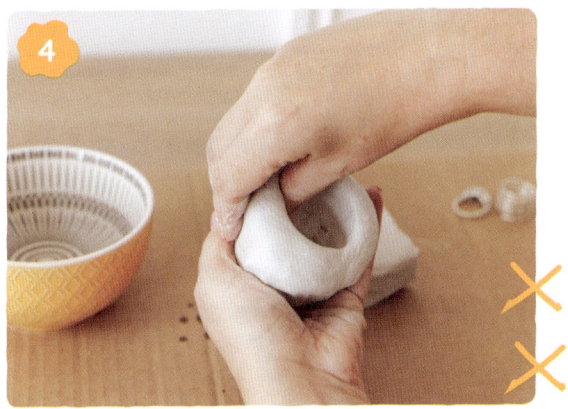

8. Once you have finished shaping your pinch pot, set it aside to dry completely. It depends on the type of clay used and the size of the pot, but for a pot this size using air-drying clay you are looking at around 24 hours of drying time.

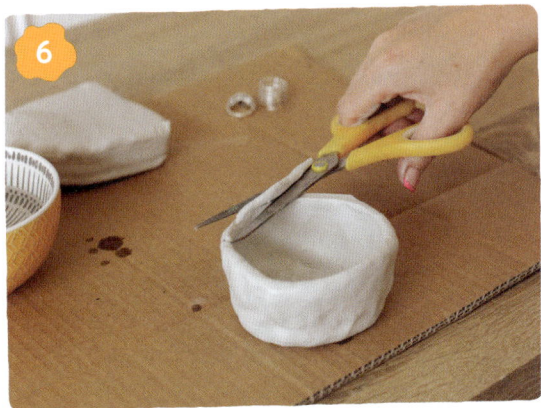

TIP: Cover your pot with a bowl or tupperware box to prevent it from drying out too quickly and cracking.

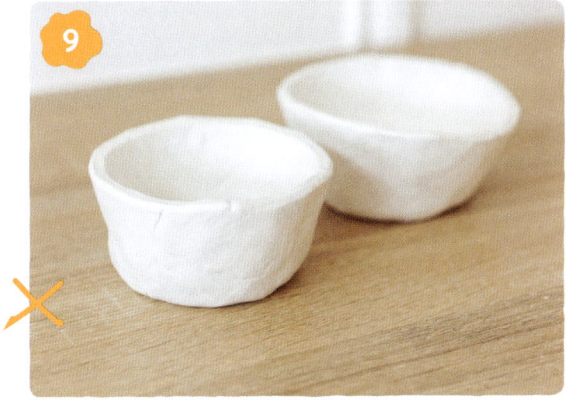

9. Once your pot is completely dry, you can paint!

10. Add a varnish or lacquer to make your pot more durable, if you wish.

⊕ Pinch pots are a great introduction to making pottery and can be made with minimal materials and equipment. They offer endless opportunities for creativity and experimentation, making them a fun and accessible project for beginners and experienced potters alike.

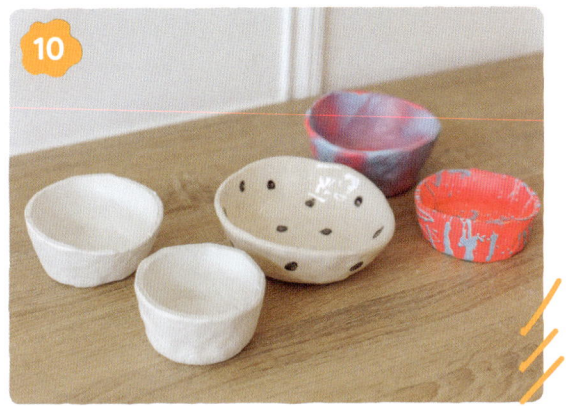

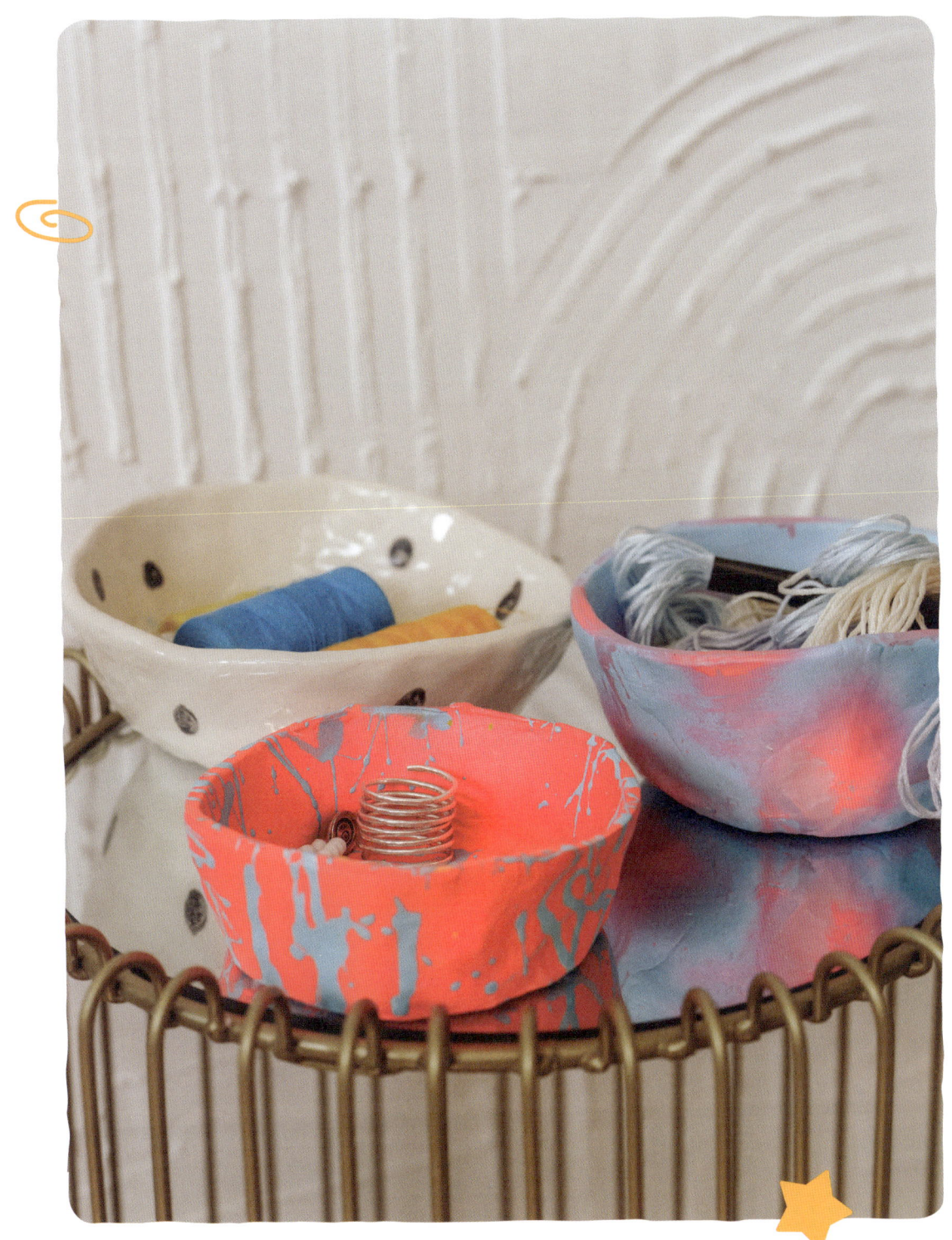

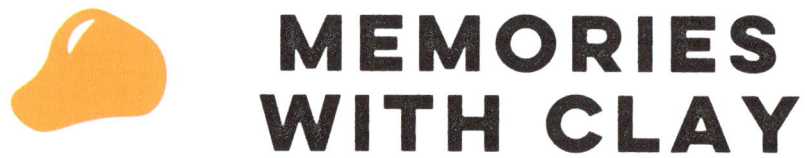 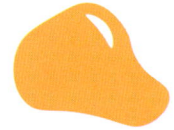

MEMORIES WITH CLAY

Creating with clay has so many wonderful benefits for our mental health. Its tactile nature makes it a great medium for reducing stress and tension, and in fact it's often used as a form of therapy. Art and in particular clay therapy is said to stimulate the brain, allowing past memories to resurface, cognitive ability to develop and new memories to form. There is also the added bonus that clay is very versatile. I've used clay to create so many wonderful things including jewellery, pinch pots and treasured keepsakes.

Sean was the life and soul. He was the joker and he had loads of mates. He was the sociable one and I was shy and quiet. I didn't find it as easy to make friends as he did.

Waving goodbye

The day we buried Sean was the day I literally waved my friends goodbye. Hundreds of people attended Sean's funeral. I remember feeling very small that day; the scale of the day overpowered me, the emotion, the people and the performance of it all. Performance may not be the correct word ... but as a child I felt part of something unknown, not real to life; it was like I was playing a part. Although

it was a formality, we had a job to do, we had to do him proud. Family, friends, parents, teachers – it seemed everyone played their part.

The funeral service was held at All Saints' Church, the church where we had both previously made our first Holy Communion, a much more joyous occasion but still as theatrical; I've always found church services to be this way.

The day of the funeral was a long one. We went from the church to the cemetery, from the cemetery to the wake. It was on the way to the wake, sitting in the funeral cars, that I waved goodbye to my friends.

The car drove past my friends who were making their way home from the church with their parents. They stood and watched the funeral cars pass, and in that moment they waved to me and I waved back. My relationship with them was different from that moment on. It was no one's fault but I was the girl whose brother had died. They didn't know how to act around me, they didn't want to upset me, and I just wanted normality.

I do believe I've struggled with building lasting relationships since then. I crave security, a guarantee that they won't leave. But no one can give me that.

This year at the young age of 40 I went on my first holiday with friends, a four-day trip to Nice in France with a circle of people I call my friends. I'm unsure if they realize just how much it meant to me. I love us as a group; we are all widely different and oddly the same. We all have our own quirks and a story to tell, we are all creatives who see beauty in the world that surrounds us.

When I spend time with them, they charge my battery, they value me, and I feel the best version of myself when I'm with them. There's no competition, no judgement, just support. I know, how

special! Is this what I've been missing out on all these years?

The holiday was beautiful on many levels and it created memories I will cherish for ever. Of course, while I was there I treated myself to a couple of little mementos as reminders of the time we spent together. As a result I am now the proud owner of a pen that looks like a baguette and a ring that turns my finger green!

It's usually little things like key rings and the universally popular collector's item, the fridge magnet, that people bring back from holiday as keepsakes. It's not so much the trinkets themselves, but more what they represent and the memories they evoke that make them valuable.

My mum has got a thing for fridge magnets, something that had always baffled me, but recently I too have started to see the attraction. I'm sure this must be a sign of old age …

What do you get when you cross a key ring with a fridge magnet? A clay keepsake, that's what!

Let's make some.

CLAY KEEPSAKES

You can't deny our universal fondness for little trinkets, so here we're going to make our own. I'm going to make a little star in Sean's honour, something I can hang in my studio and on the Christmas tree.

In a bid to keep this youthful, I've steered clear of the fridge magnets. However, this craft can easily be adapted to a fridge magnet if, like me, you've started to see their appeal!

YOU WILL NEED

★ **Air-drying clay** – you can buy the clay in small and large bags. You will need a handful for this project.

★ **Rolling pin**

★ **Cookie cutters** – stars, hearts and circles are great for all-year-round projects. Try Christmas trees, bunnies and pumpkins for seasonal projects.

★ **Knitting needle/pencil**

★ **String/ribbon/wool**

★ **Wire**

★ **Bowl of water** – always handy for shaping the clay when it starts to dry or cracks appear

★ **A glass board** or **plastic mat** – or another smooth service to work on

★ To decorate: paint, paint pens or permanent markers, decorative papers or photocopied photographs, letter stamps (these are great for adding names, dates and significant words) and magnets.

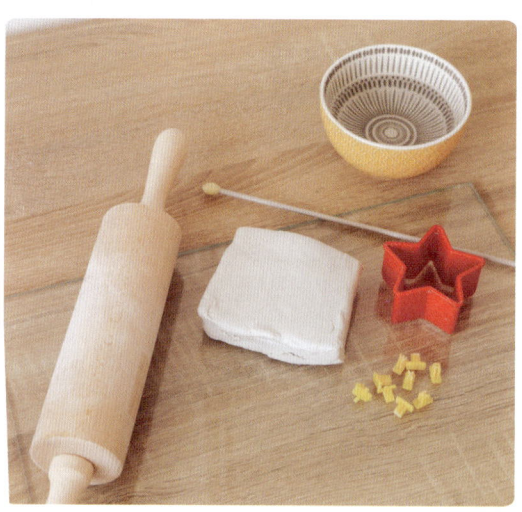

HOW TO CREATE A CLAY KEEPSAKE

1. Grab a small handful of clay and mould into a ball.

2. Roll out the clay using a rolling pin and cut out your chosen shapes with the cookie cutters.

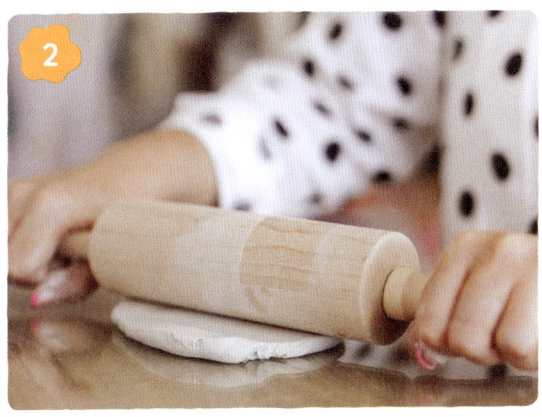

3. Remove the excess clay from around your shape and mould back into a ball; you can use this for your next ornament.

4. I'm adding Sean's name to my star. If you wish to press letters into your clay, now is the time to do it with your letter stamps.

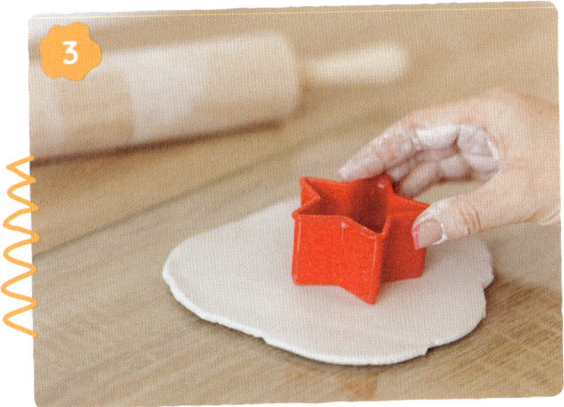

5. Using your knitting needle or pencil, create a hole in your clay shapes. If you're having trouble lifting the clay off your surface, you can use the wire to loosen it by sliding it under the clay.

6. Set aside to dry. This will take around 24 hours.

7. Once dry, you are free to decorate by painting, drawing or even decoupaging! I've used photographs of Sean and me when we were younger. See the decoupage picture frame craft on pages 119–20) for a step-by-step method.

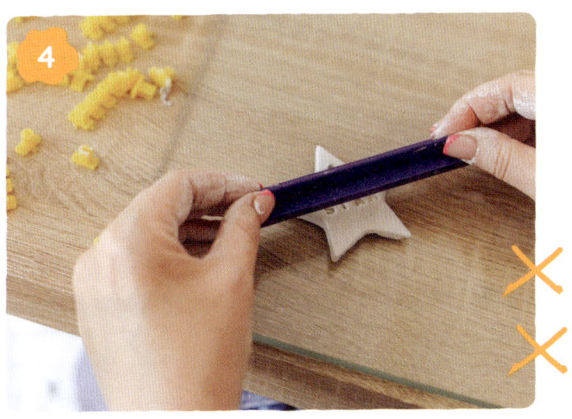

This is a fun and simple activity for the whole family, especially for the holidays as you can make lots in one go. These keepsakes make perfect gifts. They are ideal for remembering special moments and precious people. In fact, I'm just off to print the photos of my trip with my friends to make some more!

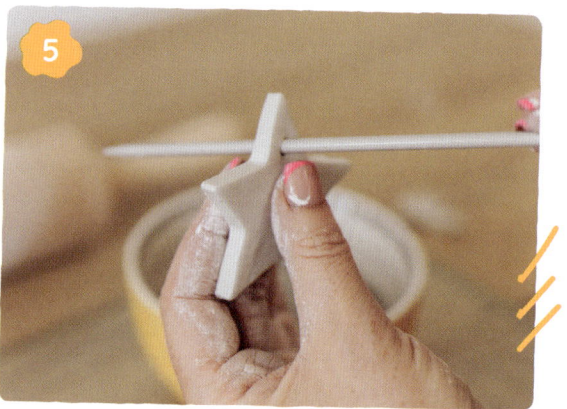

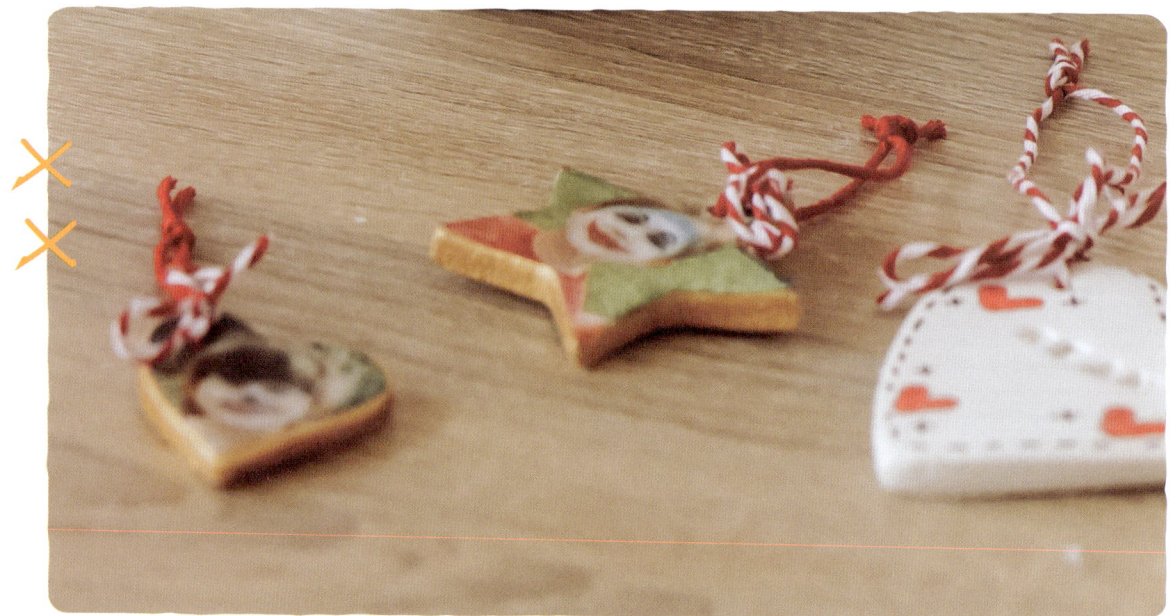

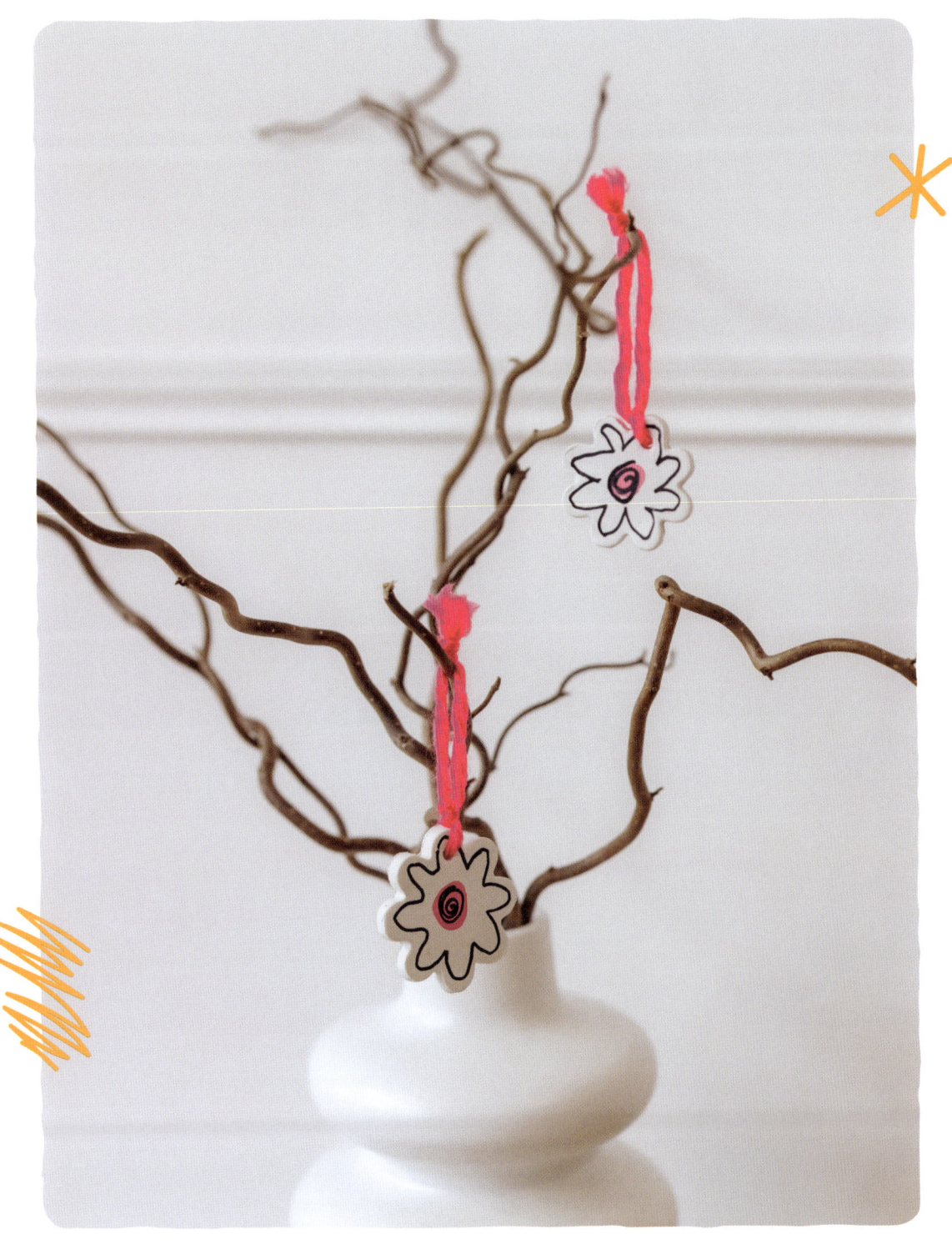

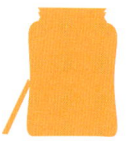 # TRASH TO TREASURE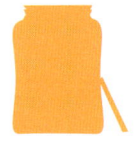

It's tough for me to say, but during my depression I saw myself as trash. I felt worthless and weak, stupid and ugly, inside and out. I don't remember the day my value returned; it crept up on me. My self-esteem grew as my small healthy habits developed into daily routines.

Now as a craft enthusiast, I see the value and potential in many things. The truth is, recycling is great, but reusing is even better! It's cheaper, more sustainable and can lead to effective resource management. So, if something can serve another purpose, then it should.

During those dark days, I neglected myself and my self-esteem plummeted. I felt as though I wasn't worthy of putting the effort into myself. The sadness consumed me, leaving me with no motivation to engage in regular daily practices such as showering, brushing my teeth and washing my hair. I couldn't be bothered, and I didn't see the point. I didn't want to go anywhere or see anyone, so why did it matter whether I was clean and well presented?

I started to hate myself and my body. I only saw the negatives. Luckily, those days are behind me now and I no longer feel worthless, weak or stupid. However, even today, all these years later, I have my hang-ups about my body and the way I look. It's sad to think that most of us feel this way about ourselves at one point in our lives. Depressed or not, it would seem that we are now more self-critical and less satisfied with our appearance than ever. Feeling unhappy with our body image can have a range of negative effects on both mental and physical health.

Building resilience

I know it's easier said than done, but it's important we are doing everything we can to protect ourselves and our loved ones by building stronger, more positive body images. And I believe this starts at home. We need to celebrate ourselves more, exactly as we are now,

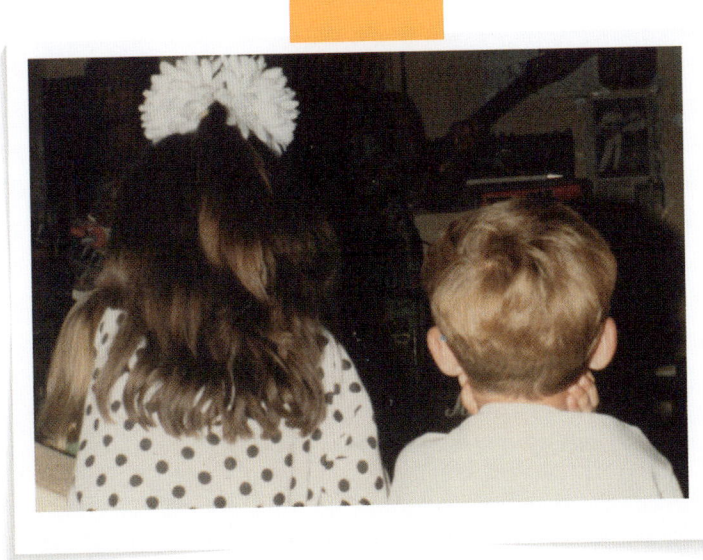

be kind to ourselves and treat and treasure ourselves.

It might sound trivial but some pampering can do us the world of good. Even during my darkest of days, a reluctant soak in the bath did lift my mood, if only for a short time. Doing this regularly created a healthy habit. I started to take pride in my appearance again, at least most of the time.

It was the same with my creative routine: allowing time for myself and my creativity played a huge part in learning to value myself again. Taking the time, however little, out of my day to create, always boosts my mood.

Glow-ups

I've always been quite resourceful, which has a lot to do with my creativity but more to do with my lack of funds and constant strict budget. Since leaving uni I have predominantly been self-employed. I started my business from scratch with very little money, so I've got used to making the best of what I have.

I would say this is where my love for upcycling came from. I keep a lot of stuff that "will come in handy one day". And most of the time, it does! I love making something from nothing, taking tired, redundant items ready for the trash and making them useful again, giving them a new lease of life, a "glow-up".

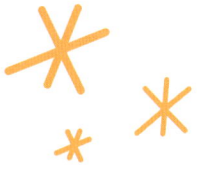

GLOW UP YOUR NICK-NACKS

We're going to turn our nick-nacks into painted personalities with a practical purpose. Glow-ups often relate to our appearance, but to glow up your mind, behaviours and attitudes has got to be the best glow-up of all.

Through my creative routine I've managed to turn my mindset around, add a little light to the darkest of days and relieve my depression. Just like the items I upcycle, my creativity has given me my own glow-up.

I think it's important that everything has a glow-up from time to time. A refresh is great for giving our homes and our things a new lease of life too. You've heard me talk about revamping clothing and furniture but it doesn't end there – you can turn any trash into treasure with a little time, some imagination and of course a splash of paint.

This is a pretty easy craft that doesn't involve much skill. I've made cake stands out of plant pots, lamp bases out of tea cups, and here I will show you how to make a desk tidy out of a jam jar!

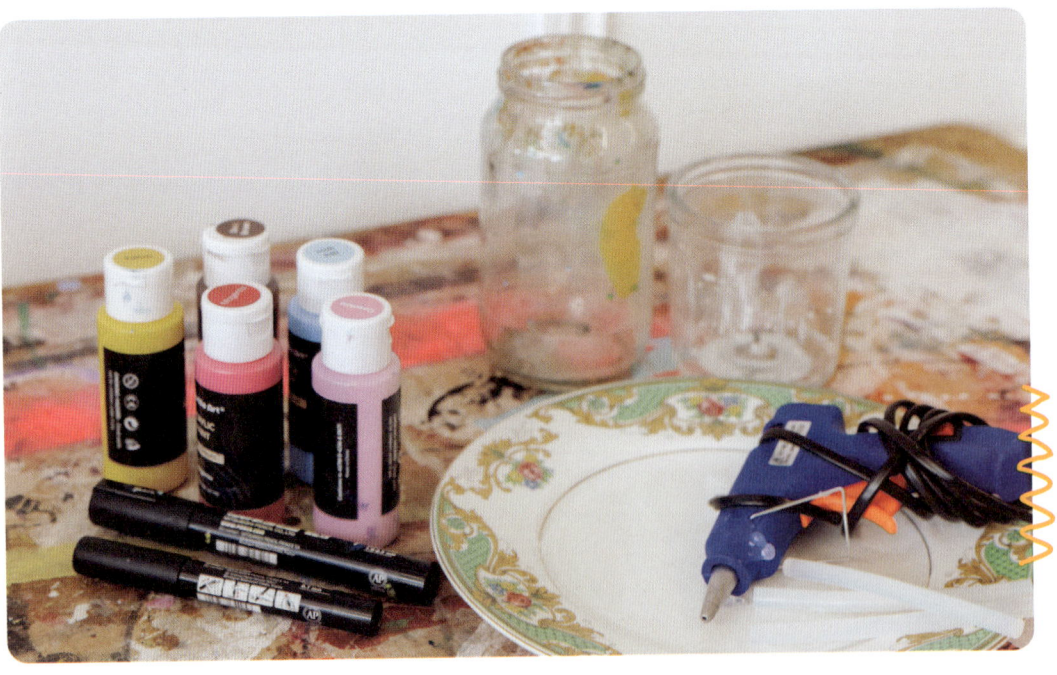

YOU WILL NEED

★ **Nick-nacks** – such as a small collection of broken or discarded crockery, glassware or jam jars

★ **Glue gun** or super glue

★ **Primer**

★ **Pencil**

★ **Paint brushes**

★ **Paint** – acrylic paint, chalk paint or household emulsions are ideal

★ **Jar of water**

★ **Paint pens** or **marker pens** – for drawing on the details

★ **Clear varnish** or **lacquer** (optional)

LET'S GLOW

1. Gather your nick-nacks.

2. Play around with stacking them until you find the best composition.

3. Glue them together using a glue gun or super glue.

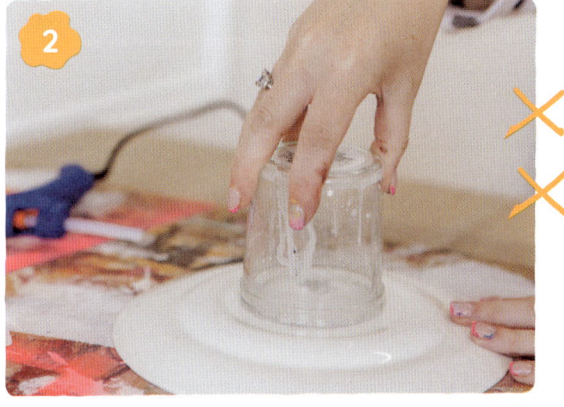

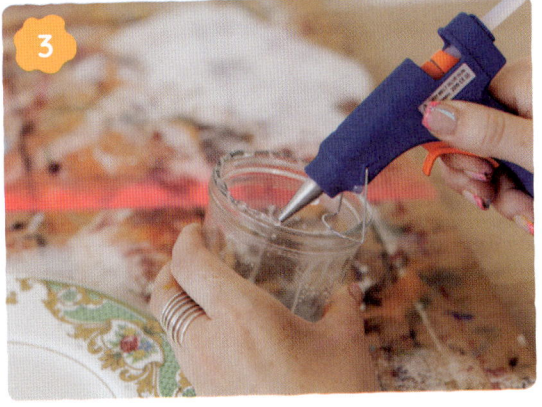

WARNING: Glue guns are hot and super glue is toxic, so all children must be supervised by an adult. Adults, you need to be careful too – I've had many burns from a glue gun, and they aren't fun!

4. Allow the glue to dry. This shouldn't take too long, both types of glue work almost instantly.

5. Cover your nick-nacks with primer. This will give you a better surface for painting. The paint will adhere to the crockery or glassware more easily and be much more durable.

6. When the primer is completely dry, mark out your chosen design with a pencil. I've decided to transform my trash into people. I will give them names and backstories and everything. This one is a version of myself who has had her own glow-up … She will be known as Queen Gemma.

7. Fill in your design with paint.

8. Leave to dry.

9. To make your glow-ups extra durable, you may wish to seal with a clear varnish or lacquer.

You will now have your own little crockery character, complete with a hand-painted personality, just like Queen Gemma. This is a creative, cost-effective and playful activity that is great for all ages and abilities, showing that broken and damaged items can still be beautiful and useful!

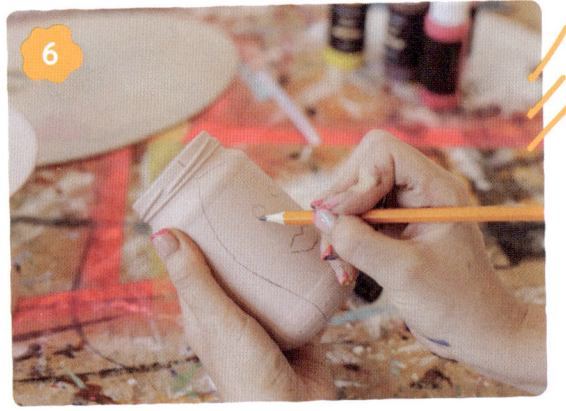

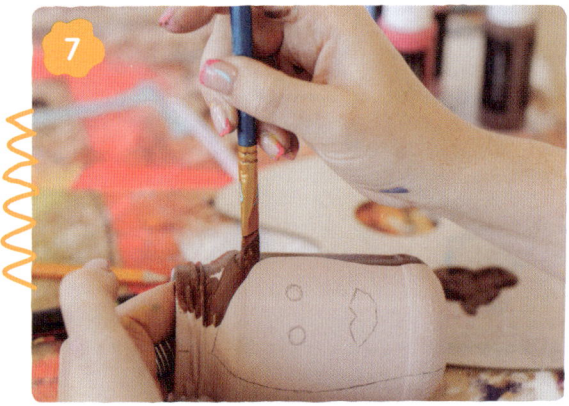

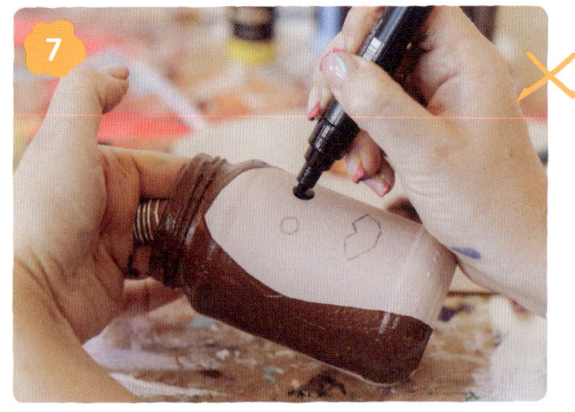

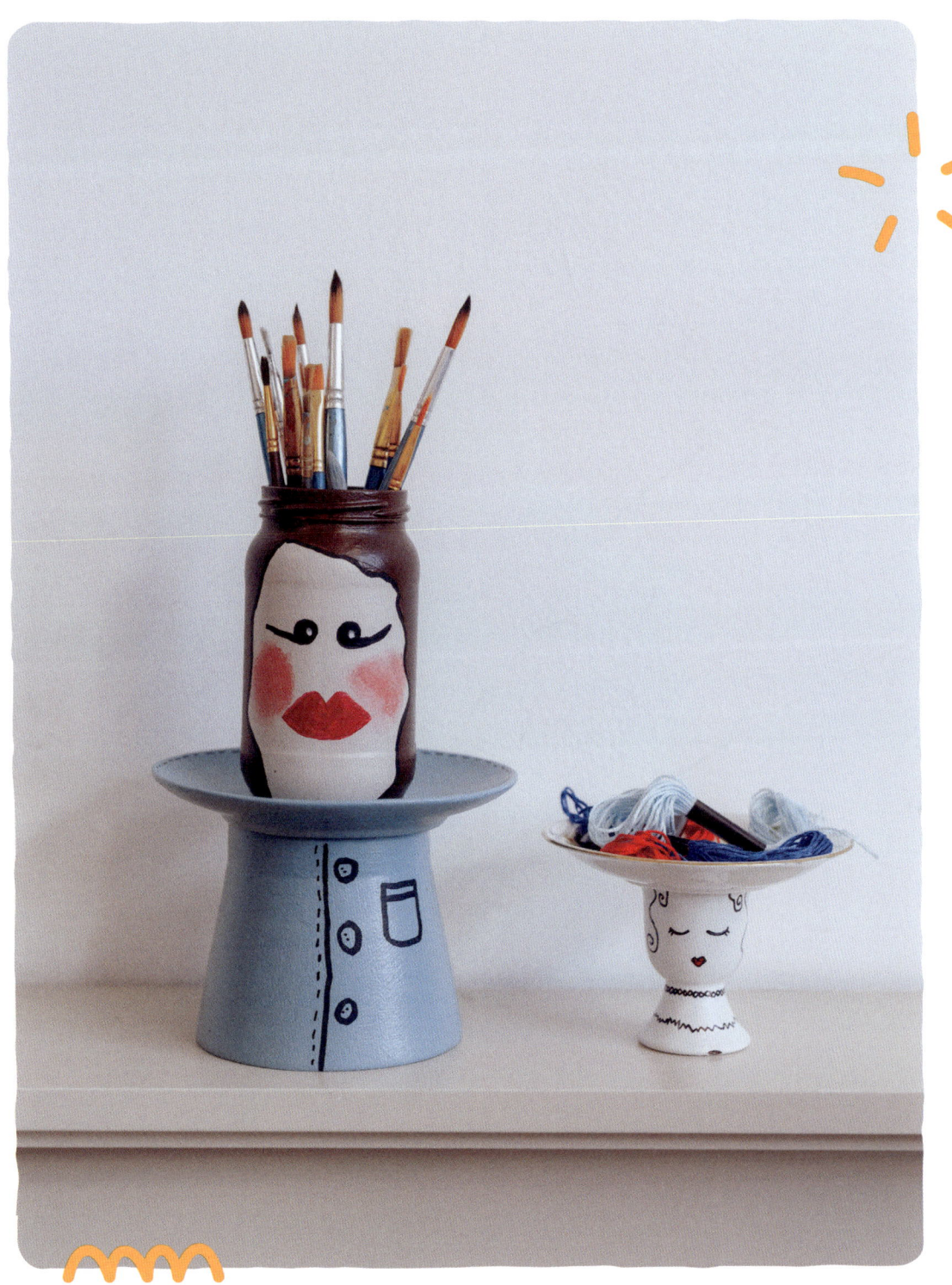

THE ART OF KINTSUGI

Mending and repairing something physically can have a huge impact on our mental wellbeing. When we fix or repair an item, whether it's a broken object, a piece of clothing or a part of our home, it provides us with a sense of accomplishment and control. Repairing and mending what's broken can help to alleviate overwhelming feelings of chaos and disorder.

Although I love to repair and mend things, I do so with a certain style, one that embraces the imperfections and celebrates flaws. Just like my own imperfections, I see scars as stories, adding character, beauty and strength.

Kintsugi, also known as "golden joinery", is a traditional Japanese art form and philosophy that involves repairing broken pottery by mending the areas of breakage with lacquer dusted or mixed with powdered gold, silver or platinum. The technique emphasizes and highlights the cracks and repairs rather than disguising them. Kintsugi is rooted in the aesthetic and philosophical concept of *wabi-sabi*, which finds beauty in imperfection and the passage of time.

What's broken can be mended

Heartbreak … Oh, isn't it awful! When I say heartbreak I'm talking about the end of a relationship and not bereavement. Having experienced both, I can distinguish between the two. Although there are lots of similarities, losing my brother was far worse than losing a boyfriend.

Still, it certainly isn't easy. I've been heartbroken twice so far. My first boyfriend, the guy I met in college who of course I thought was the love of my life, turned out to be cheating on me. That hurt … especially because we left Liverpool and moved to the same city and university together. I didn't eat or sleep properly for months. It was horrendous, but I was young and soon moved on.

The second time I was heartbroken was a few years back. Now, I don't want to use this book to air my dirty laundry, so I won't be going into details, but at the time I thought this person was my future; he promised me the world and I was left with nothing. I felt alone most of the time after losing Sean and I had hoped that I'd found my person, the person that would always be there and I wouldn't be alone again. I was wrong. I had an engagement and wedding day but not the marriage or the future I'd hoped for.

Work was a struggle. I wanted to cry all the time and some days I did. The evenings were very long, plus he took my dog when he left, so I didn't even have her to cuddle. She must have missed me.

Don't get me wrong, I'm sure I had my part to play in the downfall of this relationship. Of course I'm aware of my imperfections. However, in this case I'm sending the blame his way!

Moving on

When we broke up, I felt very low, but I was determined I wouldn't go back to the dark places I'd mentally visited in the past. I told myself he wasn't worth losing myself for.

As the months went by, I started piecing myself back together, with a little help from arts and crafts, of course. Small daily projects and activities kept my hands busy, my mind focused and my home colourful, bright and beautiful. Day by day I got used to him not being around, work got easier, my concentration, appetite and sleep all came back. I cried less and my mood lifted day by day.

Yes, I still carry my imperfections and as a result of a broken heart I'm sure there are a few insecurities. I certainly have my scars to tell the tale, but they seem to make me stronger, knowing what I've overcome, and I've become a better person for it.

Today I celebrate my scars; they make me more beautiful than I was before. When I came across the concept of kintsugi, I fell in love. I've found a technique that allows me to make broken items more beautiful than they were before … just like me.

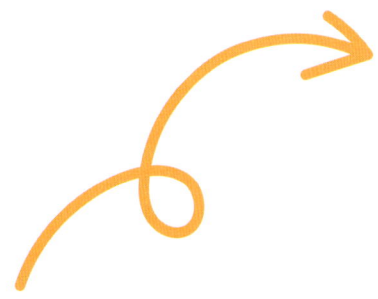

KINTSUGI PLATE

Now, this one is new to me, so we are all learning here. It's something I've always wanted to try but have never got around to. This book has given me the opportunity to do it!

A plate is ideal for beginners to kintsugi like me, but this process would also be great for larger items. I would love to try it out on a broken vase or dated lamp base. Let's get started and celebrate our imperfections!

YOU WILL NEED

★ **A broken piece of crockery** – I'm using a plate

★ **A kintsugi kit** – you can buy these online or from most craft stores. You may wish to buy all the items individually

What's in the kit:

★ **Epoxy glue** – two-part glue

★ **Gold powder**

★ **Stick**

★ **Cardboard**

★ **Gloves** – the glue is very strong so I would recommend using gloves

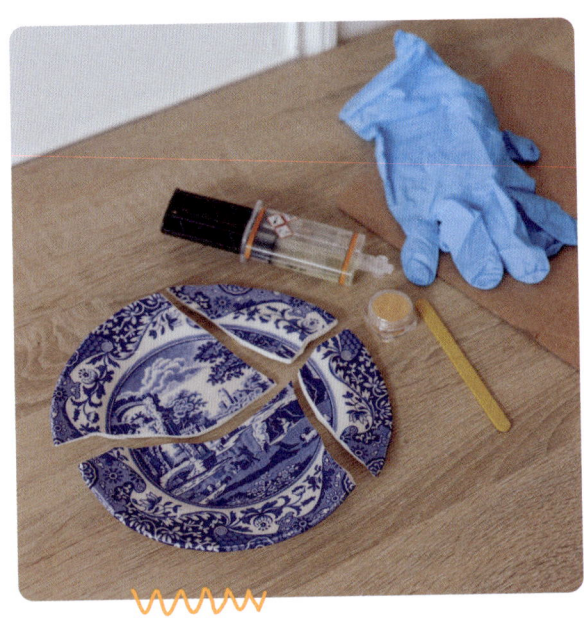

HOW TO KINTSUGI A PLATE

1. Make sure you have all the pieces for your broken item. If you don't have a broken item, you can break something intentionally. I would recommend doing this by putting your item inside a cloth or old pillowcase and banging it on a hard surface or hitting it with a hammer.

We don't want to smash our item into a million pieces. A few large pieces is easier when starting out.

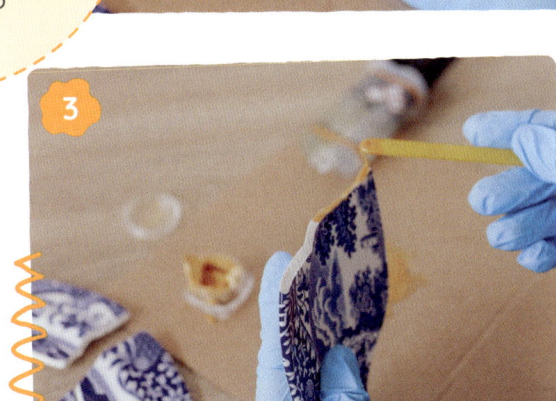

2. Mix a coin-sized blob of glue with a sprinkle of the gold powder using the stick. Too much of the gold powder will weaken the consistency of the glue, so you don't want to overdo it.

3. Using the same stick, apply the glue along the largest break and press the two pieces together.

4. Hold tightly until dry (this should only take a few minutes, but can take up to 15 minutes for larger pieces).

5. Once the glue has dried, repeat steps 4 and 5 with each piece of your plate.

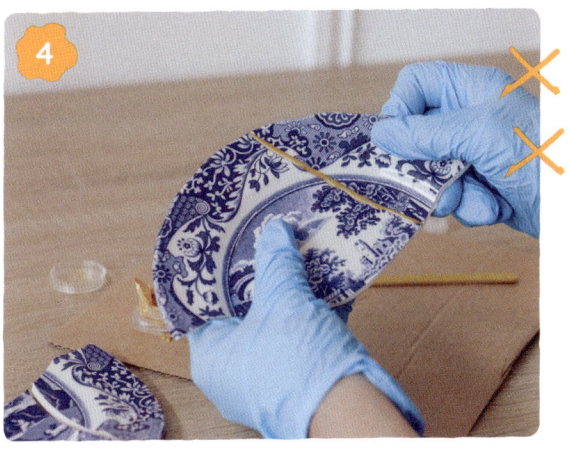

6. Piece together the larger pieces first and the small pieces last.

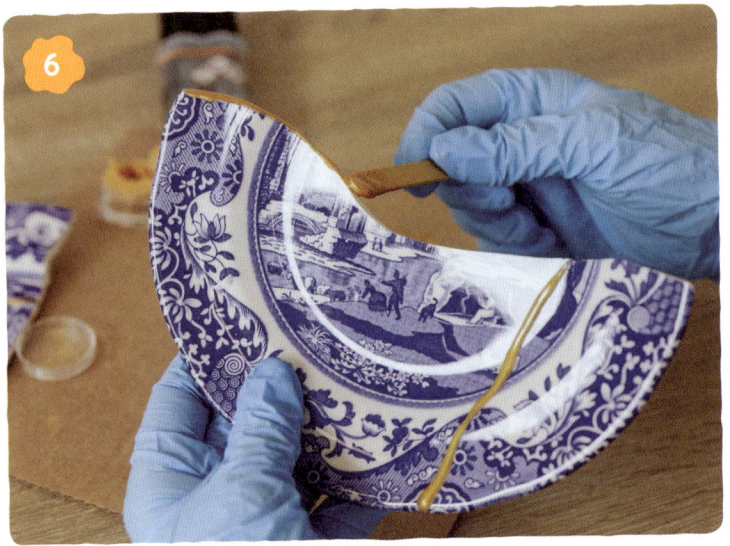

REMEMBER:
mending takes time.

I just love the idea of embracing imperfections — not only highlighting them but celebrating them.

That's exactly what this book has done for me. I'm telling my story, speaking about my darker times and celebrating them as important steps on my journey to who I am today — an author! Who would have thought?

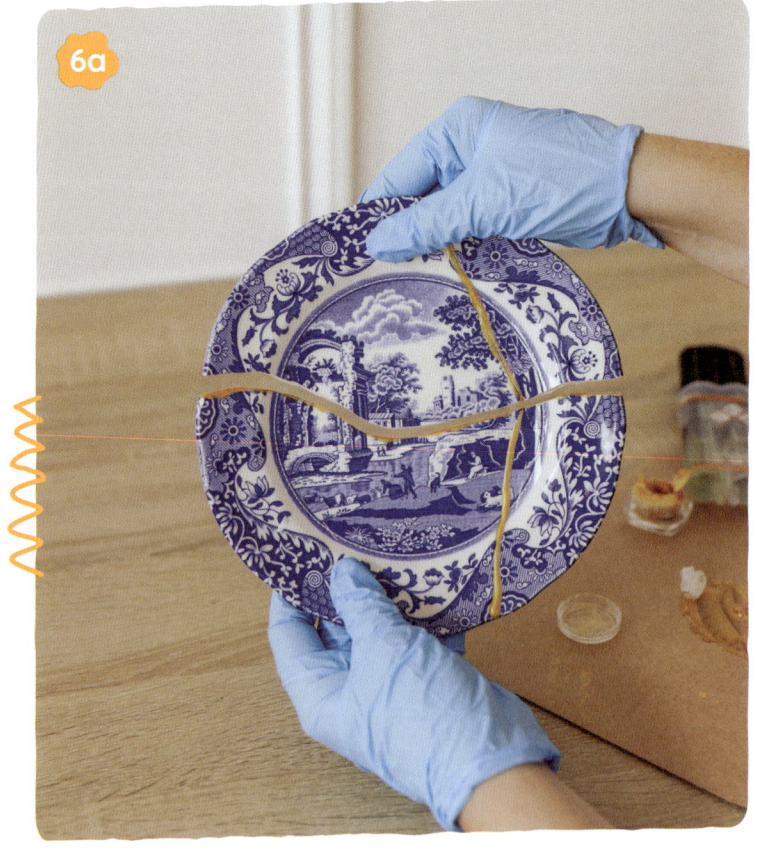

And that is it! It's a super-simple process but I've found it can be a little fiddly. Be patient when holding your pieces in place.

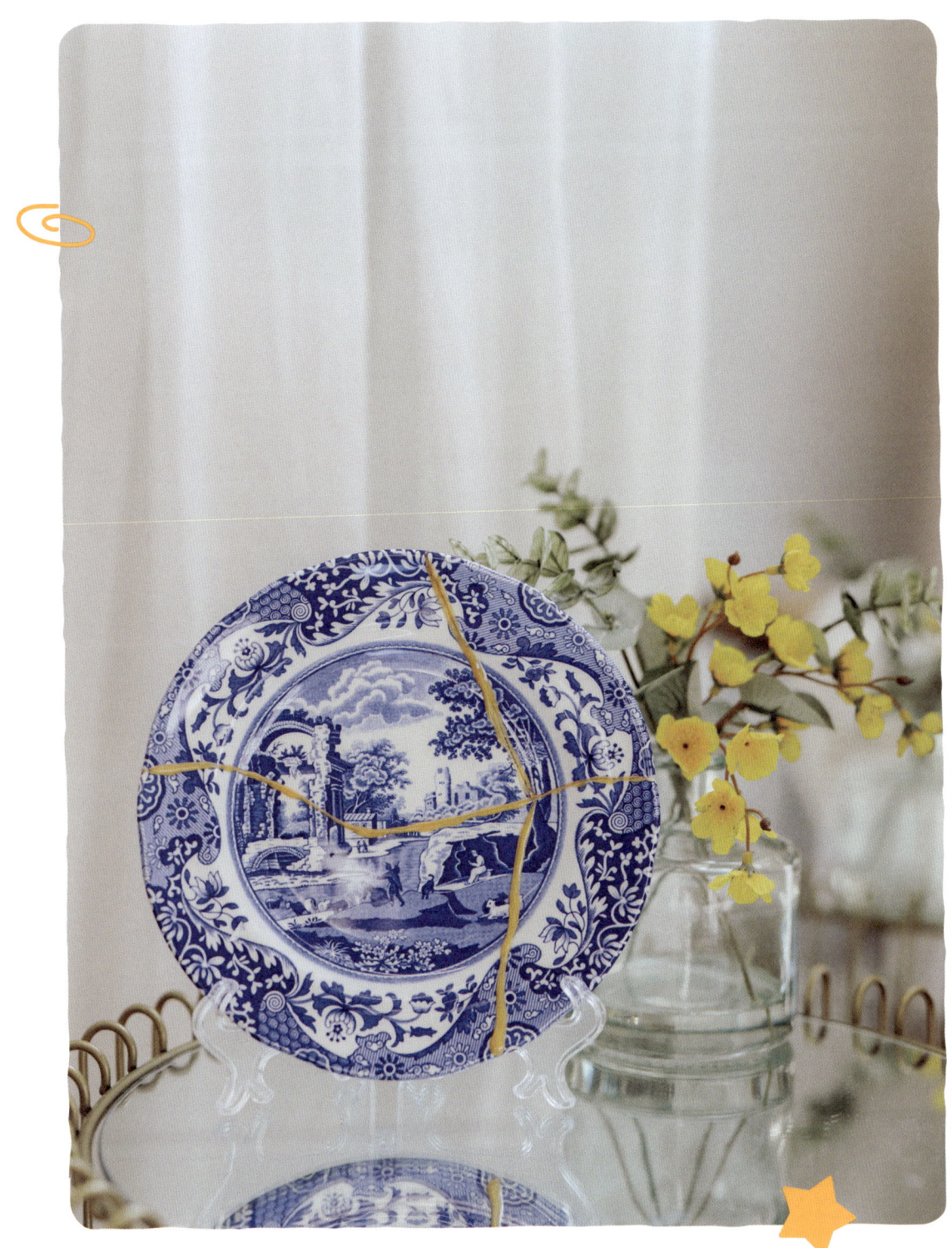

THE ART OF KINTSUGI 147

UPLIFTING UPCYCLING

Find It, Fix It, Flog It has been a turning point for me in many ways. I suppose I had a little upcycle of my own. I've grown as a person; my mindset has changed. I once shied away from a challenge whereas now I will give anything a try. It's given me confidence, boosted my self-esteem and forced me outside of my comfort zone. So I suppose what I'm trying to say here is, if an opportunity comes your way, go for it, don't let your fears and self-doubts hold you back. If you don't grab it, someone else will.

I was approached by the series producer in 2014 and was asked if I was interested in being on a TV show. The concept of the show ticked all the boxes for me: reusing, upcycling and creativity, plus as someone who had their own business it was a great marketing tool. I jumped at the opportunity and nine years later I'm still working with the team on the show and I love it. We have so much fun both on and off camera.

For those of you who don't know, *Find It, Fix It, Flog* It is a restoration and upcycling show in which the show's main presenters, Henry Cole and Simon O'Brien, scour the nation, rummaging through the barns and sheds of Britain to find languishing, preloved and unwanted items.

In each barn or shed they visit they find two items each and bring them back to the workshop to be restored, upcycled or repurposed. That's where I come in. I work from our Liverpool workshop along with Simon and Phil the handyman to bring the chosen items back to life.

Challenges and opportunities

Being on TV was never on my to-do list, so as you can imagine my first day on the job was quite nerve-wracking! I had no previous experience of being in this environment and had never been on camera before, yet here I was, mic'd up in my new workshop outfit that I had bought especially, talking to a presenter who I had never met about a mouldy barrel, with two cameras in my face. It was enough to make anyone anxious.

As much as this was a daunting experience, I am very glad I challenged myself. Working on the show has taught me so much. There has been a lot of learning on the job, as a large amount of the items Simon brings back I've never seen before. We've had everything from a birthing stool to a bird feeder, a canoe to a watering can, but rarely have I been given a perfect chest of drawers to work on. All the items come with a story and usually a problem … so my problem-solving skills have certainly sharpened over the years.

As well as the wonderful items, the show comes with a team of people, and I've been privileged to work alongside some wonderfully talented people during my time on the show. I would even go as far as to call them friends (only because they might see this).

The show has opened up further opportunities. I have presented my own episodes and visited lots of exciting and unusual places. I've been on live television and radio shows, and now look at me – I'm writing a book.

Boring to brilliant

I often get asked what my favourite upcycle has been, but there have been

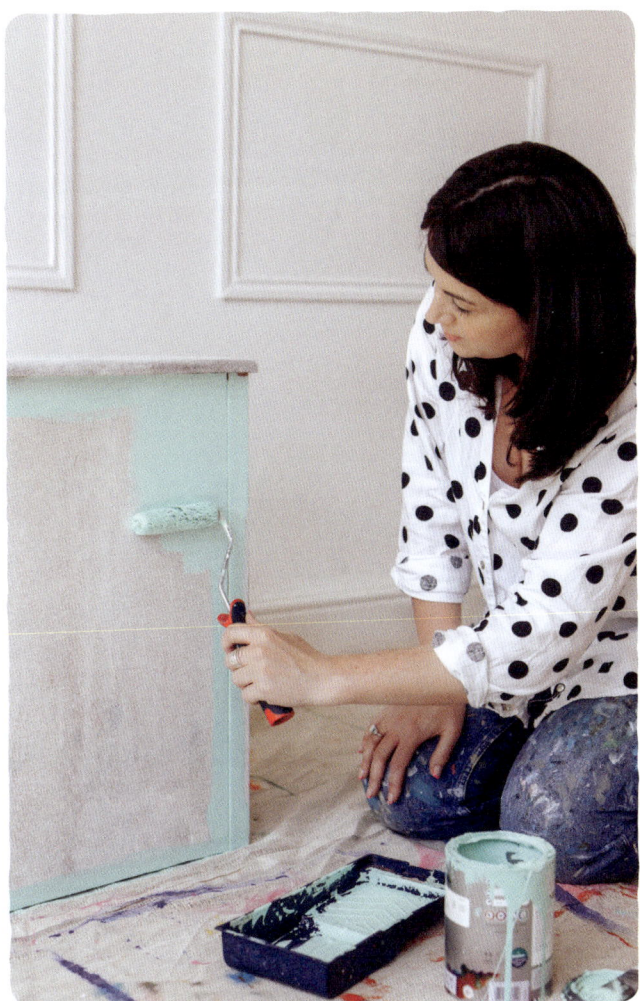

so many it's hard to remember. I did transform a rocking horse into a rocking zebra a few series back, and that was certainly a favourite. But the ones I love the most are always the colourful ones and the simplest ones, those that have been transformed with just a little TLC and a splash of paint – from boring to brilliant in a matter of hours. So let's give that a go now!

BASIC FURNITURE UPCYCLE

Sometimes starting a larger-scale project can seem overwhelming because it's hard to know where to start. However, upcycling an item of furniture doesn't have to be difficult. Sometimes a simple upcycle is all that's needed. It's the same with our mind. A series of small steps can get us started on the road to success.

Here I will take you through the basic steps for upcycling a small piece of wooden furniture. It's ideal for revamping tired items in a few hours and is perfect for items such as bedside cabinets, side tables, chairs and standing lamps. Through taking these steps with your furniture, you will also be moving forward on your path to a more positive mindset.

YOU WILL NEED

★ **An item of furniture** – I'm upcycling a small bedside cabinet

★ **Sugar soap**

★ **Bowl of water**

★ **Cloth**

★ **Sandpaper** – the grit of your sandpaper will depend on the current finish of your furniture. I find a medium grit of 120 or 80 is ideal for most jobs; however, a stubborn finish such as gloss will require a more abrasive drive such as 60 or 40 (electric sanders are much speedier, but I would only invest in one if you intend to do this often).

★ **Sanding block**

★ **Primer**

★ **Paint brush**

★ **Hoover/dustpan and brush**

★ **Roller tray** and **roller**

★ **Paint** – depending on what finish you want to go for, you can choose any furniture, wood or metal paints. Chalk paints, mineral paints and vinyl paints are all suitable. I'm using interior wood and metal paint in a satin finish.

★ **Varnish, lacquer** or **wax** (optional)

HOW TO UPCYCLE A CABINET

1. It's always a good idea to remove any fixtures or fittings before you start, such as handles or hinges that you don't wish to get paint on.

2. Give your item of furniture a good clean with sugar soap. This will get rid of any built-up grease or grime that you may not be able to see.

3. We are going to assume that your furniture does not need repairing. However, most small repairs can be carried out with wood glue or wood filler.

4. While cleaning, if you spot tiny little holes in your furniture, don't go any further without treating it for woodworm. Woodworm is common in old furniture and if left untreated can spread to other wooden items in your home. It's easily treated, so do this first.

5. Sand your furniture. As we intend to paint it, we only need to do a light sand. A keyed surface is much easier for the paint to adhere to. For ease on larger surfaces, wrap your sandpaper around a sanding block. When sanding, sand in the direction of the wood to avoid damaging the wood.

6. When you have sanded down your furniture completely, give it a good

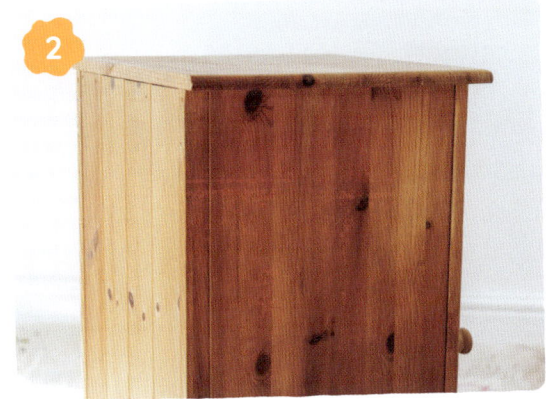

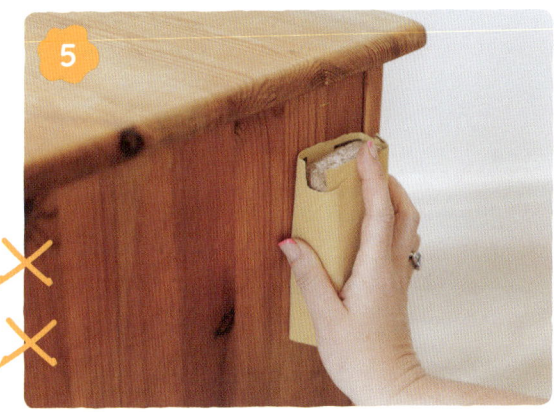

dust over; use a hoover or dustpan and brush if needed. We don't want any dust getting in our paint.

7. It's prime time. Apply a primer to your furniture with a brush for the more intricate areas and a roller for the larger surfaces. Primer will prevent any stains or imperfections coming through to the paint and it will also help to give your paint an even coverage.

8. Furniture primer tends to come in two shades – white and grey. I choose which to use depending on my paint colour. For lighter colours I go for white and for darker colours I choose grey.

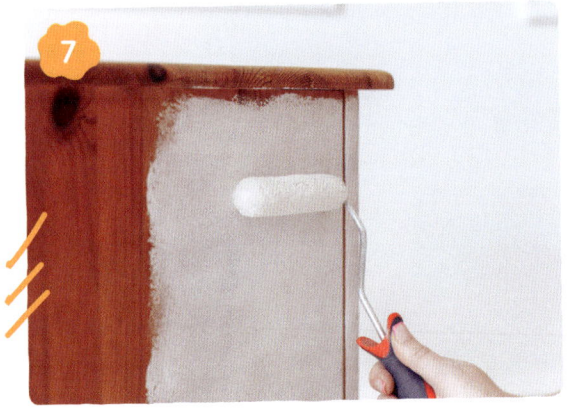

9. When the primer is completely dry, it's time for the transformation. I find this the most fun part, getting the colour on! Just like the primer, apply your paint to more intricate areas with a brush and larger surfaces with a roller. You may need to build up your colour with two or maybe three layers, depending on your colour. If so, allow each layer to dry completely before adding your next.

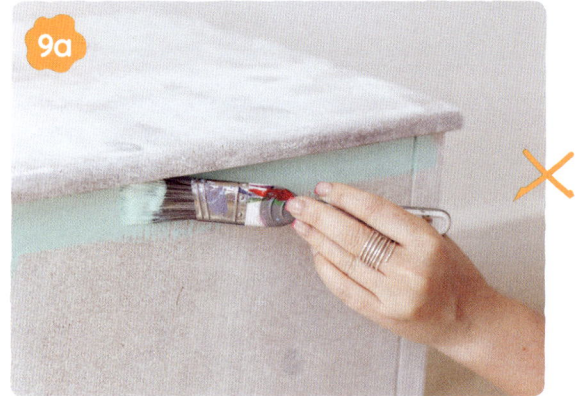

10. I've used a satin finish paint, so there's no need to add a varnish, but you may wish to add a varnish, lacquer or wax over your paint to protect it.

11. When everything is dry, you can put your fixings back on if you took them off at the beginning.

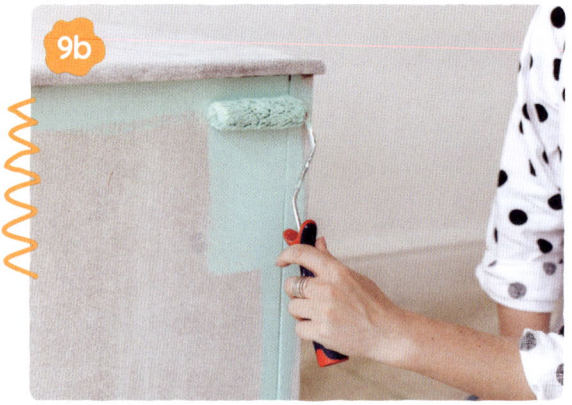

Paint and varnish take time to cure so although your furniture will be touch dry in a matter of hours, it's always a good idea to leave your newly revamped furniture a few days before using. Some paints can take up to four weeks to cure. If you use your item before the paint has had time to cure, it will be prone to scratches and scuff, so do be careful.

There's nothing better than upcycling an item of furniture and then using that item in your own home. It's a permanent reminder that transitions don't always have to be hard and that you can be anything you want to be. Even when you're tired and broken, with a bit of TLC you will become a better you.

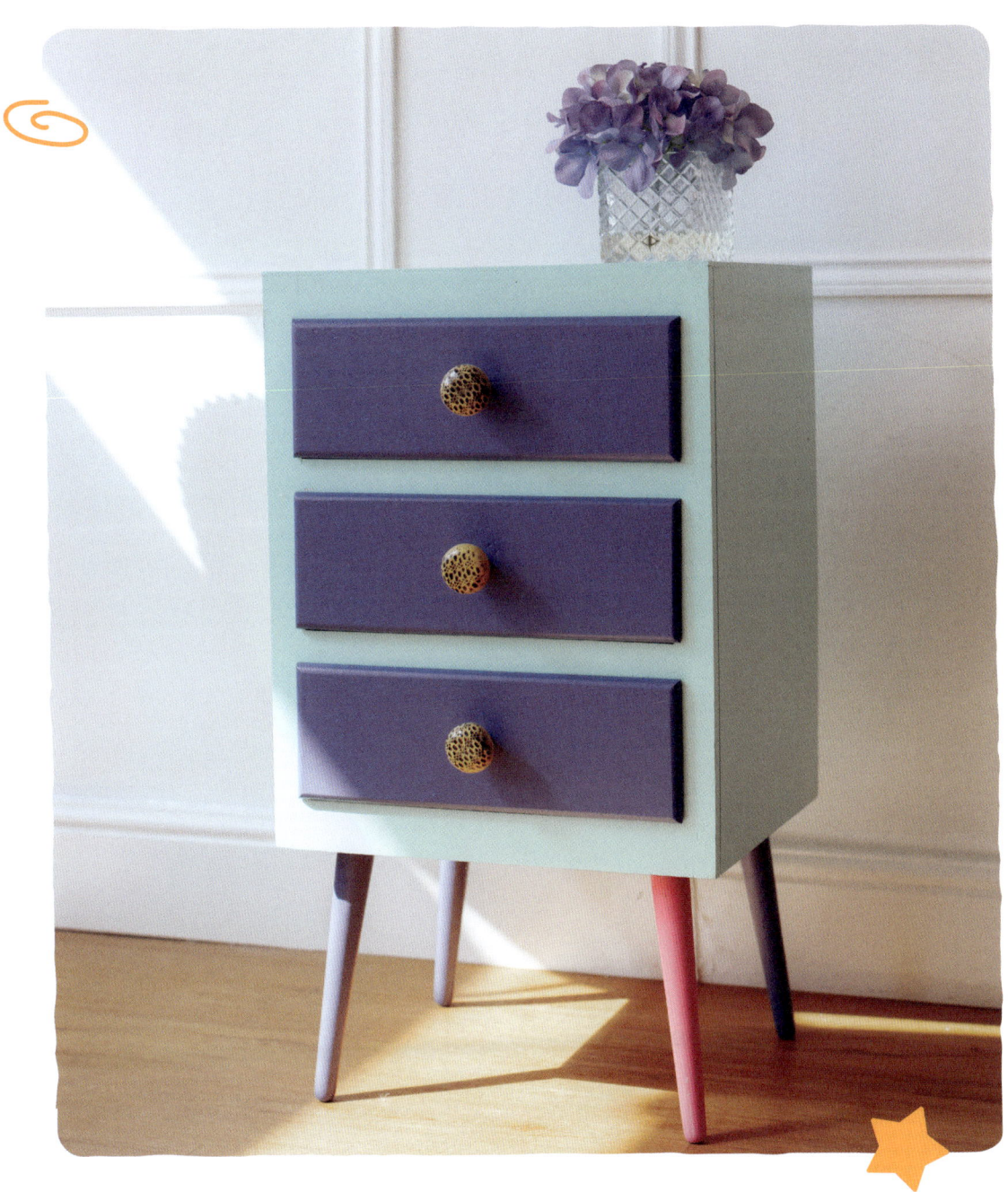

UPCYCLING WITH UPHOLSTERY

For me, comfort is key. If I'm comfortable then I'm at ease with myself. Yes, there is something to be said for getting out of your comfort zone. But right now, we're staying comfy. Upholstered furniture can help to create physical comfort in our home. Upcycling with upholstery can bring us emotional comfort too because we're looking after our mind through a creative routine.

So what is upholstery? Upholstery refers to the covering of furniture, specifically chairs, sofas and headboards with fabric. Nowadays, there are two types of upholstery: traditional and modern. Traditional upholstery uses classic methods such as hand stitching, springing and tacking and materials such as horsehair, cottons and wools that have been around for centuries. Modern upholstery embraces contemporary techniques such as machine stitching and stapling and materials such as synthetic foams and wadding.

Upholstery is a skill. It's certainly not easy and can take time to master … I'm still learning. Personally I find modern upholstery easier and the materials more accessible. I love adding upholstery to my upcycles whenever possible. It's great for adding colour and pattern through fabric. If you choose the right fabric, you can really add the wow factor to your upcycles.

Rest days

On days like today it's a challenge to get anything valuable done at all. I just want to sit or sleep or watch rubbish telly. I think the correct terminology is procrastinating.

I don't want to work, I don't want to write or respond to emails, I don't want to prepare for workshops or network; I definitely don't want to pay the bills, do the dishes, hoover the bedroom; it's a firm no to the food shop, and the gym is absolutely out of the question (but I never want to do that, not even on my best days). In fact, it's been a few days now where I have achieved very little. My mind can't seem to focus and all I want to do is sleep.

Over the years I have come to realize that due the nature of my work, the fact that I work for myself and the emotions that come from my work – not only my emotions but the emotions of others – although it can be incredibly fun, it can also be exhausting. It can be stressful.

The importance of downtime

I now understand the importance of resting both mentally and physically. Rest helps reduce stress and anxiety, improving overall mood and mental wellbeing. Adequate rest enhances memory, decision-making skills and concentration. It replenishes energy levels, ensuring you can perform daily activities effectively. Rest supports a healthy immune system, helping the body fight off illnesses. It allows muscles to

repair and grow after physical exertion, reducing the risk of injury. So, rest is vital and we all need to make sure we are enjoying some downtime.

I struggle to rest, although I am getting better. I'm always busy and feel guilty when I'm not doing something. I especially find it hard to rest when there is something that needs to be done. I can rest easier if I've completed my to-do list or finished a project I'm working on. I've got a holiday coming up, so it feels like a race against time to get all my jobs done before I go. I want to be able to thoroughly relax and unwind.

Maybe I'm getting old, but the idea of having everything on my to-do list finished so I'm able to completely relax sounds like perfection to me!

If, like me, you struggle to rest and you're looking for an excuse to have some downtime, then maybe you should upcycle your own chair to do just that! I've got the basics down so I'm going to share them with you.

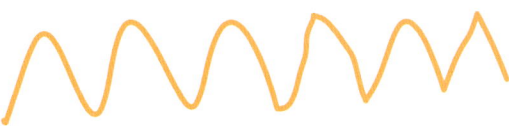

PULL UP A CHAIR

- -

Upholstering a chair and mending your mind may seem very different, but there are interesting parallels between the two. In essence, they both involve processes of restoration, personalization and improvement, each aimed at enhancing overall wellbeing and functionality.

Here I'm going to upholster a chair that I've upcycled. It's fine as it is, it's colourful and it's functional, but I want to push it further. I see this chair as a representation of myself: I've worked hard to get it to be ok, but now I want it to be confident and brilliant.

Through fabric, colours and pattern, this chair will reflect my style, my growing confidence and self-worth. The upholstery on the chair is like the icing on the cake … Let's do it.

YOU WILL NEED

★ **A chair** – a wooden dining room type of chair, ideally with no padding or cushion

★ **Upholstery foam** – this comes in a variety of thickness to suit all projects. I'm using 5cm/2in-thick foam for this chair.

★ A **pen** or marker

★ **Scissors** – you'll need sharp fabric scissors for cutting the foam

★ **Spray adhesive**

★ **Wadding** – choose the flame-retardant varieties for your projects

★ **Staple gun** – my staples are 10mm

★ **Fabric** – it is advised that you use flame-retardant fabric for all at-home projects. There are also protective sprays available if your chosen fabric is not flame-retardant.

Your seat may be separate to your chair, in which case your upcycle will be much more straightforward. Regardless of whether your seat is attached or separate, follow these steps.

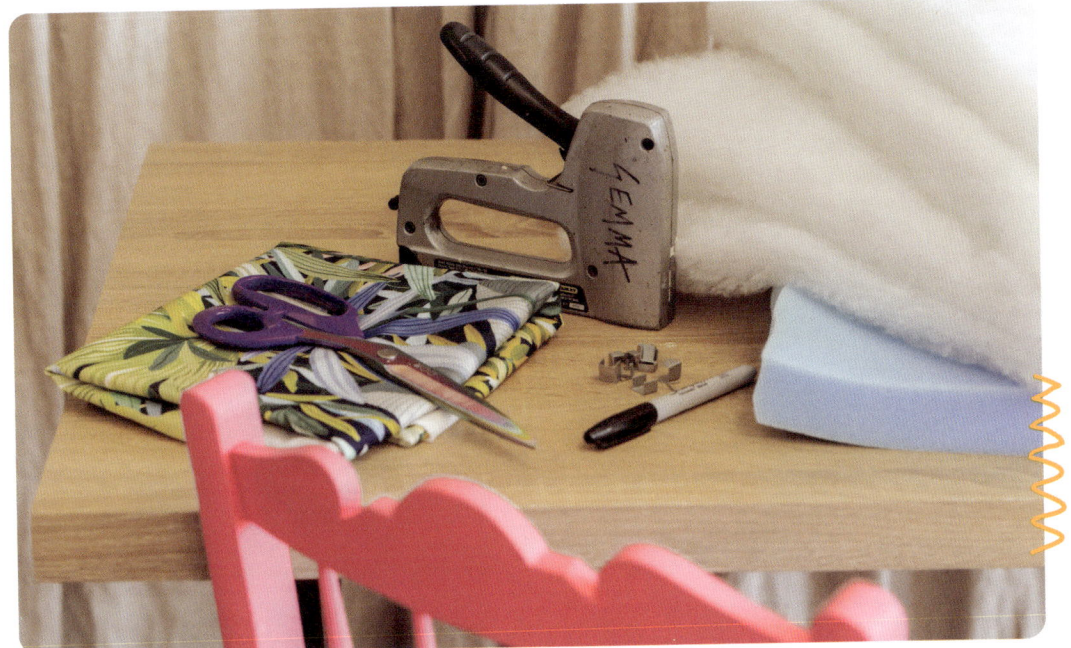

1. Cut your foam to size by drawing the seat of the chair directly onto the foam. Sharp scissors will be able to cut straight through the foam.

2. Using spray adhesive, stick the foam to your chair seat. This prevents the foam from moving.

3. Cut a large piece of the wadding and cover the foam.

4. Turn your chair upside down. I find the next steps easier if I position my chair onto the end of a table.

TIP: You may wish to follow the steps from the basic upcycle (see pages 151–2) to add a little colour to your chair first.

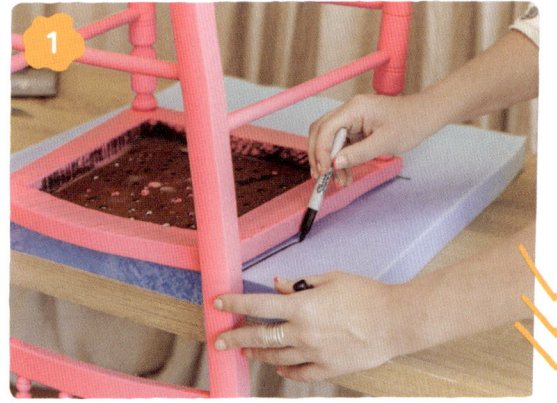

5. Staple the wadding to the underside of the chair, going around the edges and pulling it taught as you go.

6. Trim off any excess wadding.

7. Appy your fabric over the wadding and put your chair in the same position as before.

8. Staple the fabric to the chair, pulling the fabric taught as you go and folding over the edges to create a tidier edge.

9. When it comes to the corners, it gets a little tricker. Pull one side of the fabric around the corner and staple in place. You will then be able to fold the remaining fabric neatly and staple it in place.

⊕ No, there's no excuse: you've upcycled a chair, it's looking fabulous and you can't let all that hard work go to waste. So, have a seat and relax ... You've earned it.

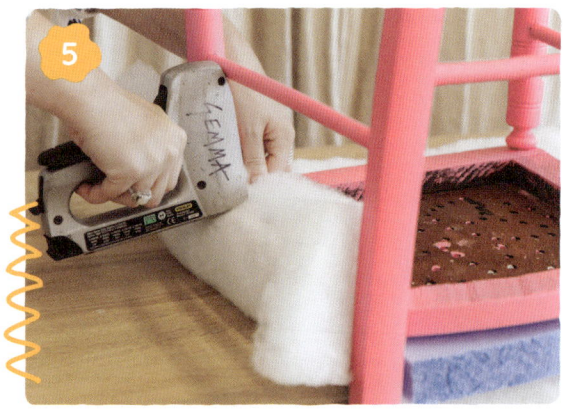

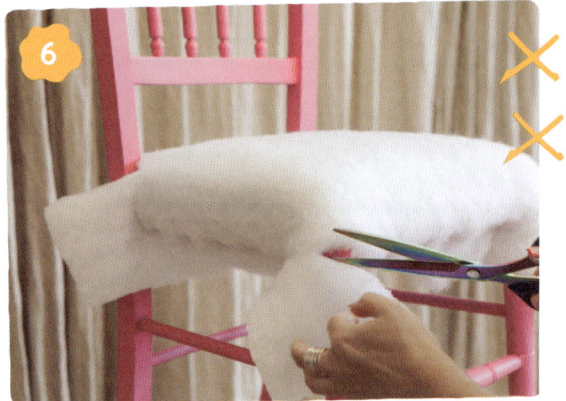

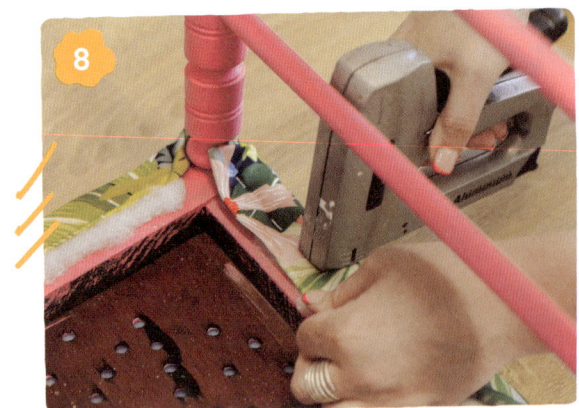

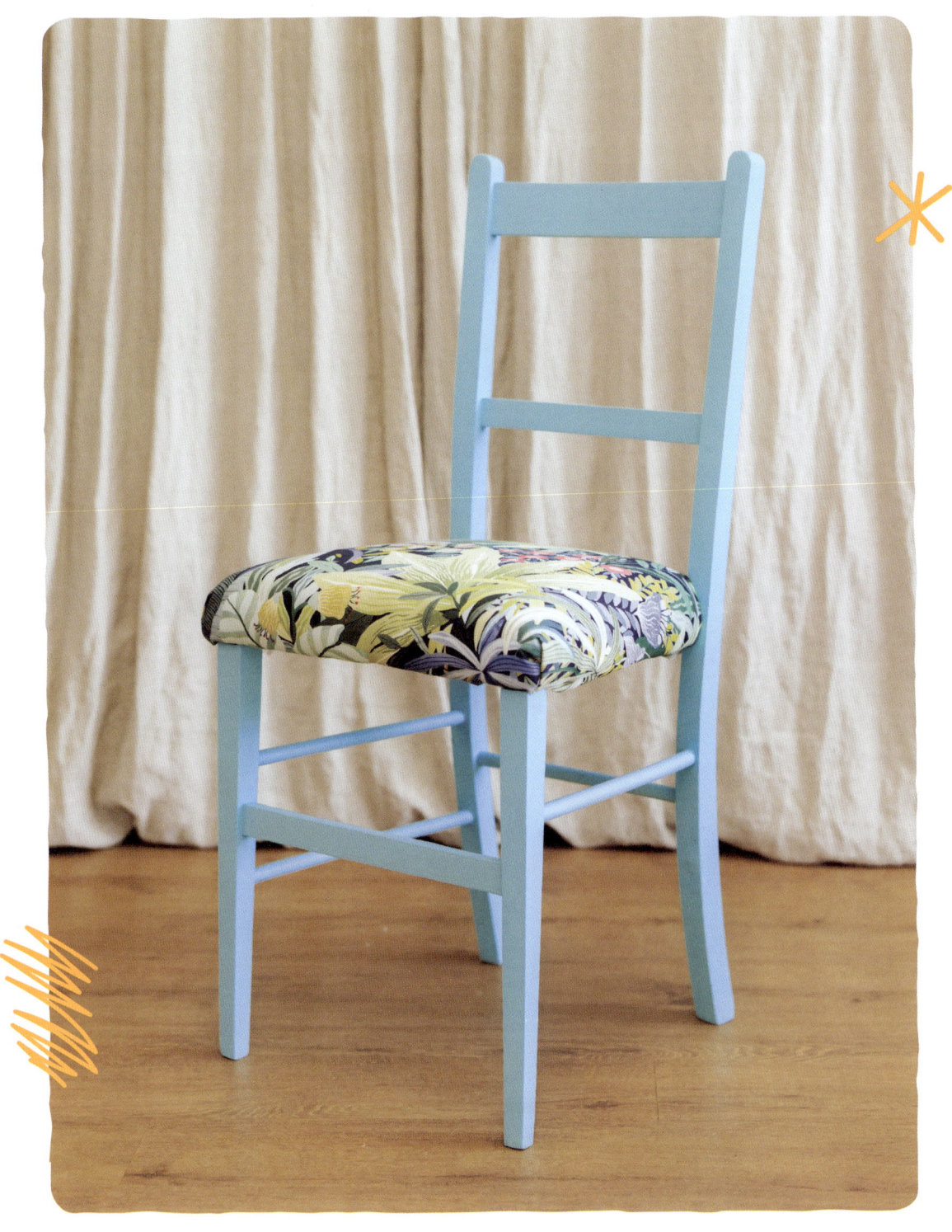

PATCHWORK DECOUPAGE

For me, there's nothing better than taking an item of furniture that was tired and unloved and revamping it into a treasured item. It reassures me that there is always hope and anything can be saved with a little love. Similarly, when we're feeling down, a bit of TLC can transform us into something strong, vibrant and valued. Granted, it might take a little more than some wood glue. But the creative process can give us a new lease of life.

Since I started filming *Find It, Fix It, Flog It*, a lot of people have contacted me with their old, unwanted furniture, and as much as I want to say "yes" to everything, I simply don't have the space to. However, if there is a story attached, I find it difficult to say no. So, a word of advice for anyone who wants me to take their furniture: lead with the sob story!

For example, a lady got in touch with me whose mum had recently passed away and she was selling her house. No one in the family wanted the furniture, so she asked if I could use any of it. Of course, I couldn't say no. Among other things, she had an old school desk, a dressing table and one of those spindle standing lamps. I was in love, and what made these items more special was that they came with a story. She shared memories of doing her homework at the desk and her mum getting ready for the bingo sitting at her dressing table. I think it's the stories that I fall in love with.

Memories

When someone passes away, a family is often left with a lot of belongings, and sometimes we are talking about a lifetime's worth. A family often prefers to hold onto smaller items such as clothing, photographs, nick-nacks and books, as they don't take up so much space. But often the larger items of furniture are just too big to keep and end up in the tip, which is such a shame.

Furniture, just like photographs and items of clothing, holds memories, and when possible these items should be saved. My nan died of dementia when I was 20 years old. At times, she was very weak and needed bed rest. I remember my mum and I would sit next to her in bed. At the foot of her bed was a large brown wardrobe, one of those proper old-fashioned ones made up of three compartments and three doors. The middle door was a full-length mirror.

My nan would often get confused and, not realizing it was a mirror, she would wave to the people at the bottom of the bed, then whisper things about them to me. She often commented on the state of the young girl's hair – which of course was me! Although it was very sad that my nan was so ill, it did make my mum and I laugh to hear her unknowingly insult us.

That wardrobe holds those memories for me. It's part of her tale. Just like my grandad and his armchair. He loves that armchair, he's always sitting in it every

time you visit. This has got me thinking – which item of furniture is part of my story?

Cherishing unwanted items

We may inherit pieces of furniture that are not quite to our taste, or maybe don't fit with the style of our homes, but this shouldn't deter us from keeping them. There are many ways in which we can upcycle them – stencilling, painting and decoupaging, to name just a few. There are many fabulous decoupage techniques that offer stunning transformations, but this patchwork decoupage is a simple, affordable and effective method for transforming boring to brilliant.

When you upcycle an item of furniture, you are getting the best of both worlds: a cherished item that holds so many memories, and a new look tailored to your home. If you can also mentally benefit from the creative transformation process, you are winning all round.

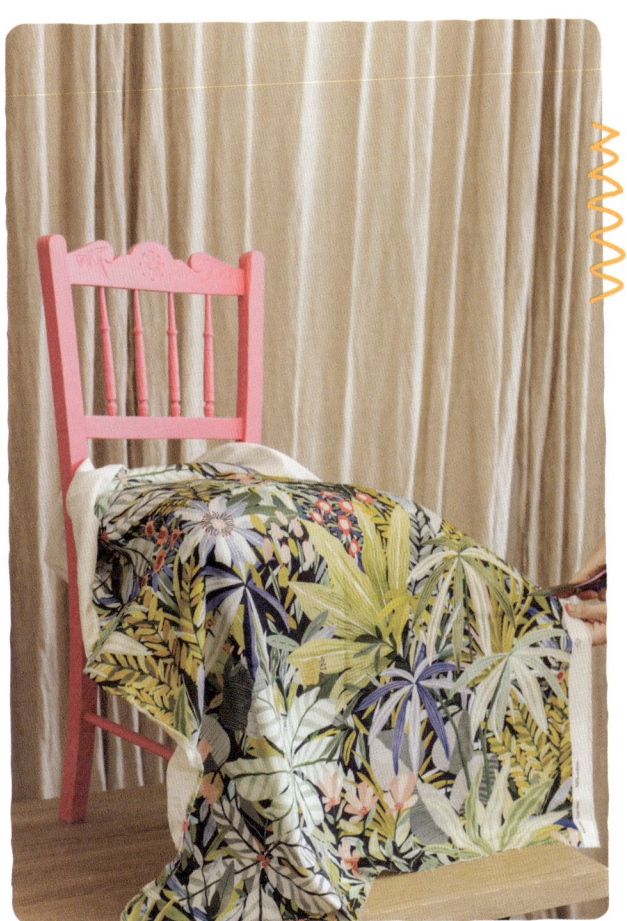

PATCHWORK DECOUPAGE TABLETOP

It's official, you've got the decoupage bug like me! This project is decoupage on a slightly bigger scale: we're going to upcycle a table.

If you're a beginner to upcycling with decoupage, I would advise that you use furniture you're not precious about while you're practising. That way, if it doesn't go to plan, you've not lost anything, and if it does go to plan (which of course it will) you've transformed an unloved discarded item and saved it from the bin. Go you!

YOU WILL NEED

★ **A table** – if you don't have a little table at home, you will be able to find one easy enough at your local charity shop, or online second-hand and preloved websites. Don't go spending huge amounts, though, let's keep this budget-friendly. Although it's great to work with old furniture, if you are struggling to find something, you could always buy a new budget table from your local discount store.

For the upcycle: (see page 150 for the complete list)

★ Sandpaper

★ Primer

★ **Paint** – a tester pot of paint should be more than enough for this project

For the decoupage:

★ **Paper** – ideally a minimum of five different types, colours or patterns. You can also use thicker papers such as wallpaper for this project, as we are working on a larger flat surface.

★ **A separate piece of paper for template**

★ **Pen** or **pencil**

★ Scissors

★ **Decoupage medium** or **PVA glue**

★ **Paint brush** – to apply glue

★ **Varnish, sealant** or **lacquer** – although this isn't important for smaller projects, it is required for this project to protect against damage

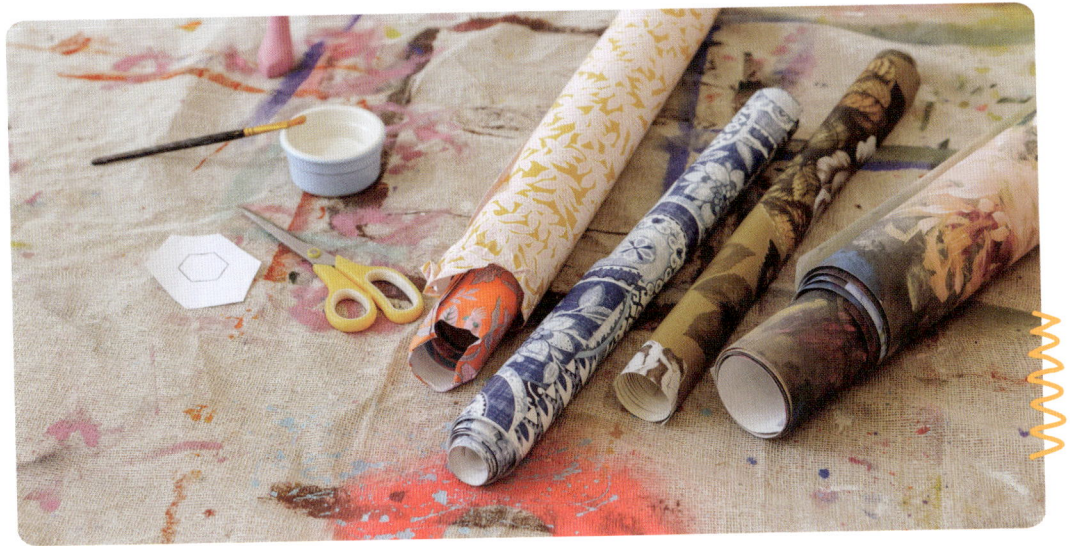

HOW TO DECOUPAGE A TABLE

If you are painting your table, follow the steps in the "basic furniture upcycle" project on pages 151–3. Once you are happy with your paint job, it's time to decoupage. Make sure your paint is completely dry before decoupaging.

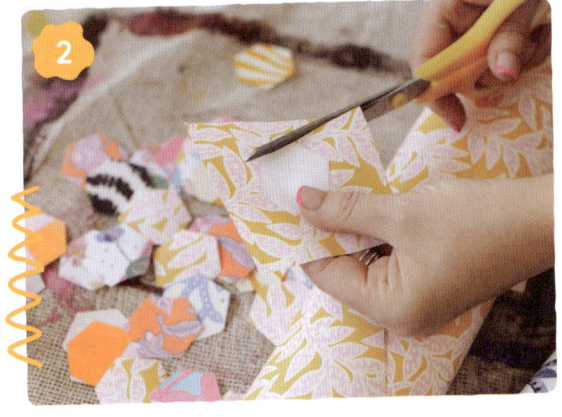

1. Cut out a hexagon template. Make it easy by printing one out, or trace off the computer screen or phone, or use the templat at the back of this book.

2. Gather your paper. Using the template, cut out hexagons from all your selected papers. How many you will need will depend on the size of the surface you want to cover.

3. When you're happy that you have enough hexagons to cover the surface of your table, lay them out. As we are aiming for a patchwork look, ideally avoid having two hexagons of the same pattern next to each other. It's at this point that it starts to look fab. You will be feeling pretty pleased with yourself, and your serotonin levels will be on the increase.

4. Let's lock that in and stick it down. Apply the glue to your brush, paste onto the table, stick your paper hexagon over the glue. Once it's in place, apply glue over the top of your paper hexagon. To clarify, you will be glueing both under and over the paper hexagons. Repeat, repeat, repeat until the surface is covered.

5. Leave to dry!

6. Once your table is completely dry, apply a coat of clear varnish. This will prevent scratches and tears in the paper and make your tabletop more durable and water-resistant.

⊕ There we have it. We've saved a piece of furniture from landfill, created a one-of-a-kind item for our home and our serotonin levels are through the roof.

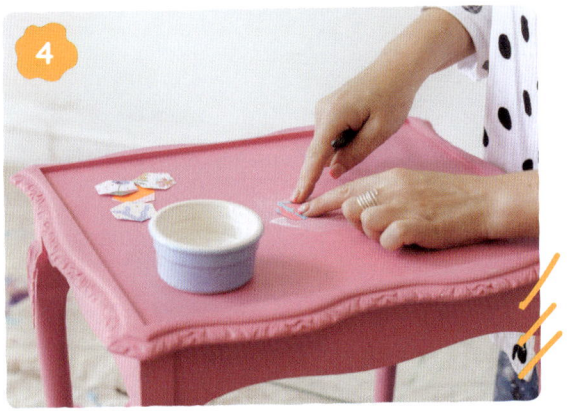

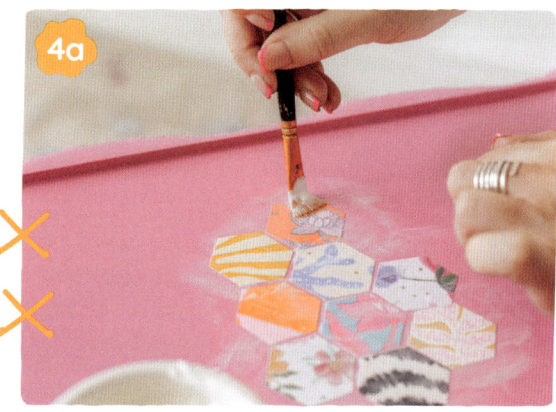

TIP: Depending on how precious you are about your table, and the papers/memories you may have used to decoupage with, you may wish to cover your decoupage with a piece of Perspex or glass. If you take a cardboard template of your tabletop to your local glazier, they will cut a piece of glass to size. Ask for toughened glass with rounded edges.

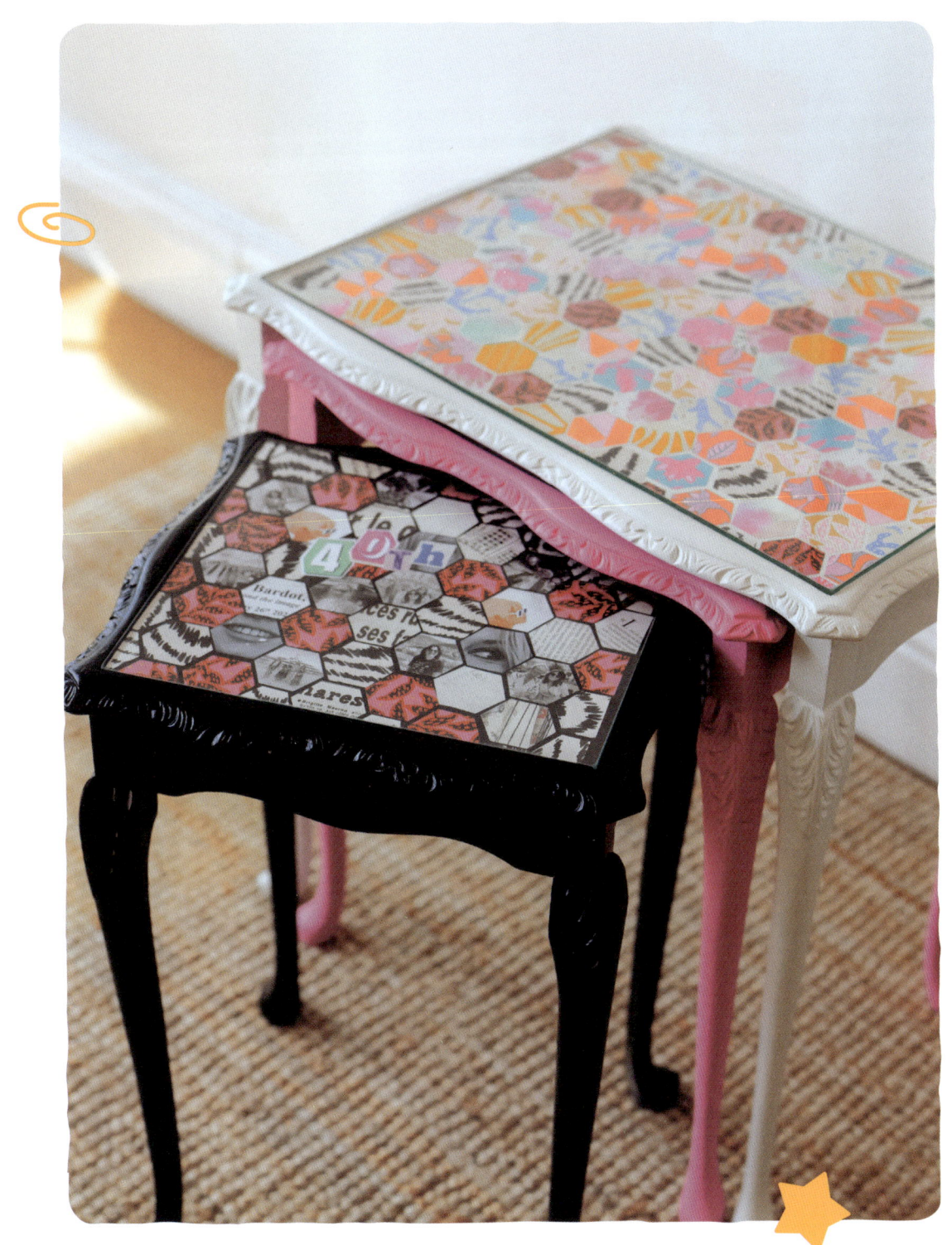

MAKE YOUR MARK

With this book, I want to encourage as many people as possible to try art and crafts as a therapeutic tool. I want as many people as possible to reap the benefits. If you think that you're not good enough to pick up a paint brush and create or that you're "not the creative type", this could be just what you need.

I've reached the age of 40 and, on the whole, I'm happy. It's been quite the journey; I've had some pretty rough times and lots of great times. I've come to realize in my wise old age that life is full of ups and downs ... It's rarely smooth sailing. It's the moments in between the extreme highs and lows that have a bigger impact on our lives than we realize.

Over the last few years, I've got to know myself better. It's an ongoing process, as I'm forever changing and developing from the experiences that come my way. However, I think I'm starting to get a clear understanding of who I am. I'm self-aware, I know my strengths and I know my weaknesses. I know my triggers, I have my fears and I have my dreams. I also have bags of energy and determination for the future.

My creative journey

I've had some pretty dark times and I'm proud to say I've got through them, maybe a little scarred but all the stronger for it. I'm sure I have plenty more ahead of me and more emotions to feel, both good and bad; however, I now feel I'm better equipped to deal with what comes my way.

I have my creativity to get me through whatever's around the corner. Art has become something that fills me with joy. When I visit art exhibitions, I often cry, not because I'm sad but because I can see so much beauty around me. I see stories, I see feelings, I see expressions.

My creations are, for me, good, bad, beautiful or ugly ... but mostly, they have got me to where I am now and I look forward to where they will take me next. They have allowed me to see beauty and potential in the small things, the imperfections and the transitions we go through.

My creative journey began with a fashion wheel when I was just a child with dreams. I then drew to be close to my brother, I painted to express myself and I upcycled to see change.

Today I have the courage to make my mark on whatever is around me without fear of judgement. I have goals that I'm working toward, I'm taking little steps and making little masterpieces as I go.

This book has been a process for me – a tough one, might I add. Since I started writing this book, I have launched Hidden Gems, a creative bereavement support group here in Liverpool, a group that supports children and young people who have been affected by the death of a child to open up and express themselves through art. Children just like I was 29 years ago. I hope that through coming to Hidden Gems the children will find a way to release their emotions and become less isolated in their emotions as they build valuable relationships with others who are experiencing similar feelings to their own.

Transformation

The final activity in this book is one of transition, of self-expression and explosive creativity. It's for you to make your mark on whatever it is you have.

I want you to imagine this item as yourself at the start of this book and, using what you've practised throughout the book, I want you to make your mark and transform this piece of furniture into you now. Hopefully a more positive, creative and colourful you.

If I'm honest, I wanted this piece of furniture to be massive. I'm talking a huge wardrobe, a garden shed or even a mural … a showstopper. But as the photoshoot for this book was in London and I travelled from Liverpool, the 200-mile journey made that a little difficult!

In an effort to have a little variety I ruled out a chair, table or bedside cabinet and opted for … a shelf! I know, not quite the scale I had in mind, but it could fit in the van and allowed me to type the line …

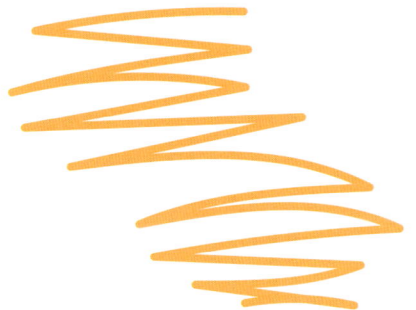

SORT YOUR SHELF OUT

This activity feels like a good ending for this book, as it combines many of the processes we've done together throughout the book:

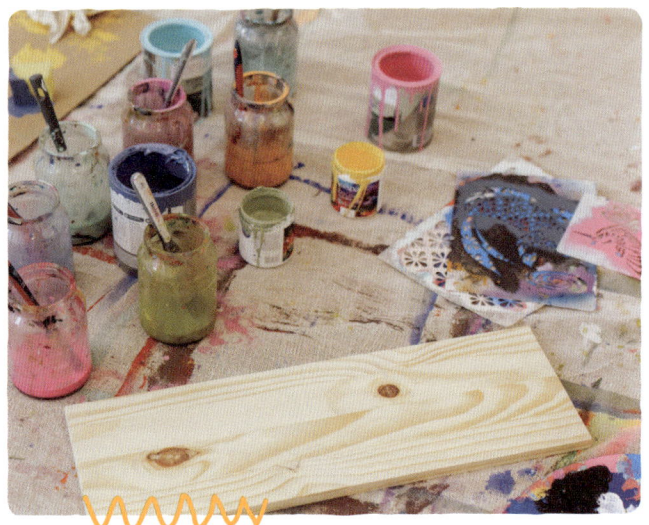

Upcycling

Revamping

Repurposing

Expressive painting

Doodling

Stencilling

YOU WILL NEED

★ **An item of furniture** – if you're following me, a shelf. I get these shelves all the time to practise paint techniques on, as it is much cheaper than buying wood!

★ **Primer**

★ **Paint brushes** and/or roller and roller tray

★ Paint

★ Stencils

★ **Paint pens** or **marker pens**

★ Oil pastels

★ Sponges

★ Spray bottles

★ **Clear varnish** or **lacquer** (optional)

★ **Drill**

★ **Drawer knobs, handles** or **hooks** if creating a coat rack like me

HOW TO SORT YOUR SHELF OUT

These instructions are for a shelf, but I would encourage you to adapt them for your alternative item.

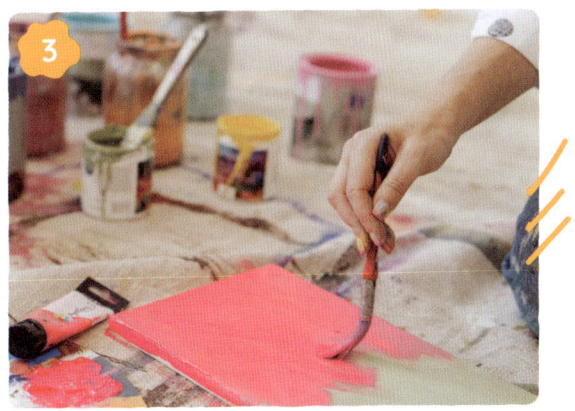

1. Make sure your shelf is clean and free from dust. Give it a light sand if needed. Mine is bare wood so doesn't require any sanding.

2. Prime the entire shelf with a brush or roller, then leave to dry.

3. When the primer is dry, paint on your background in a variety of colours; the more expressive your brush strokes, the better. Leave to dry.

4. Add stencils over your background. Leave to dry.

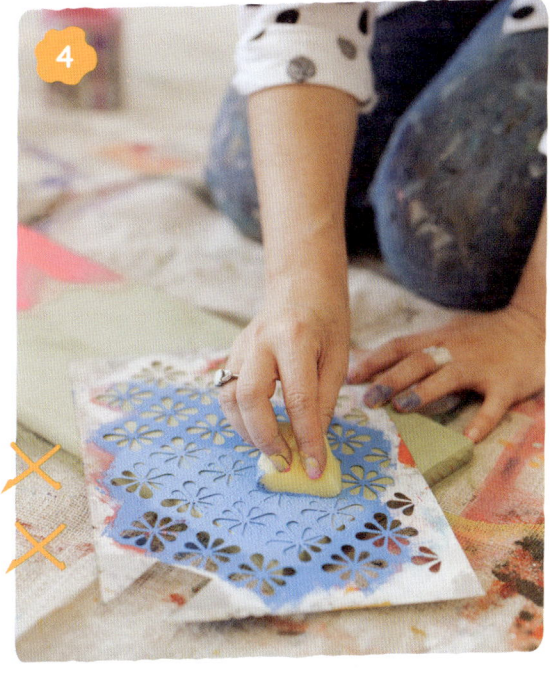

5. Add your own details to your shelf. I've sprayed on watered-down paints, done doodled with paints and hand-drawn details using oil pastels.

6. When everything is completely dry, you may want to seal it with a clear varnish or lacquer. If you have used oil pastels like I have I would recommend this so the oil pastels don't rub off onto your coats when hanging.

7. I have taken three drawer knobs that I didn't need from another upcycle project and painted them black to use as hooks for my rack. (I will find a use for everything!)

8. I measured my shelf lengthways and made sure all my hooks were the same distance apart. It is easier to find the middle, this is where your first hook will go, then measure an equal distance either side for the next two hooks.

9. I also measured from the top of my shelf to make sure the hooks are sitting in the middle of the shelf. Mark out where your hooks will be with a pencil.

10. Drill a hole for each of the markings, making sure your drill bit is the same as the fixing.

11. Screw on your hooks.

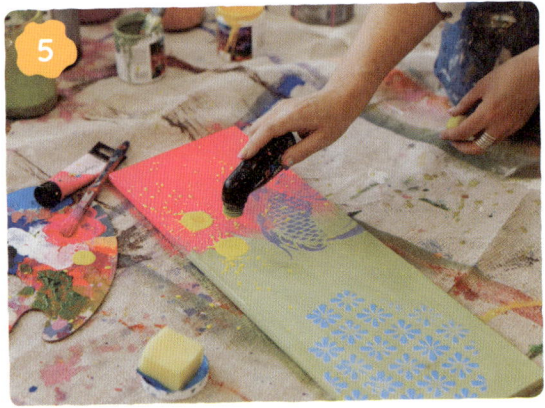

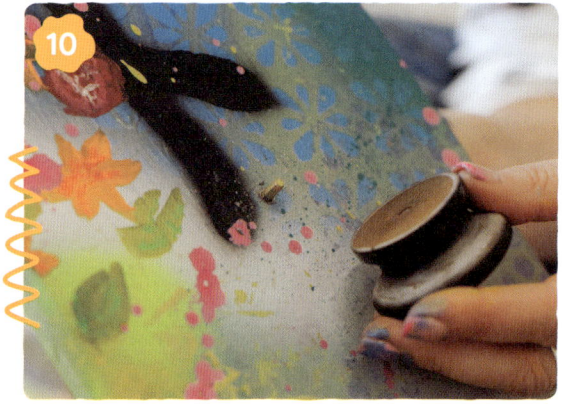

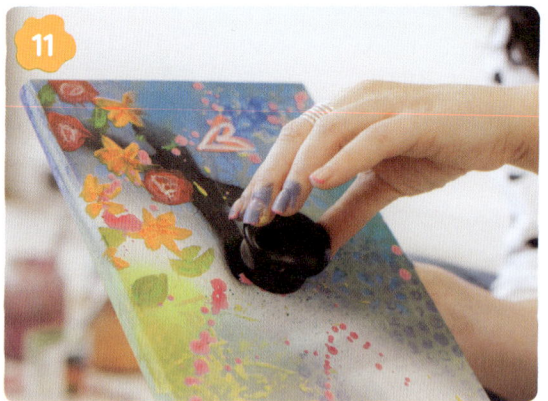

Hang your upcycled coat rack up on the wall along with any negative thoughts!

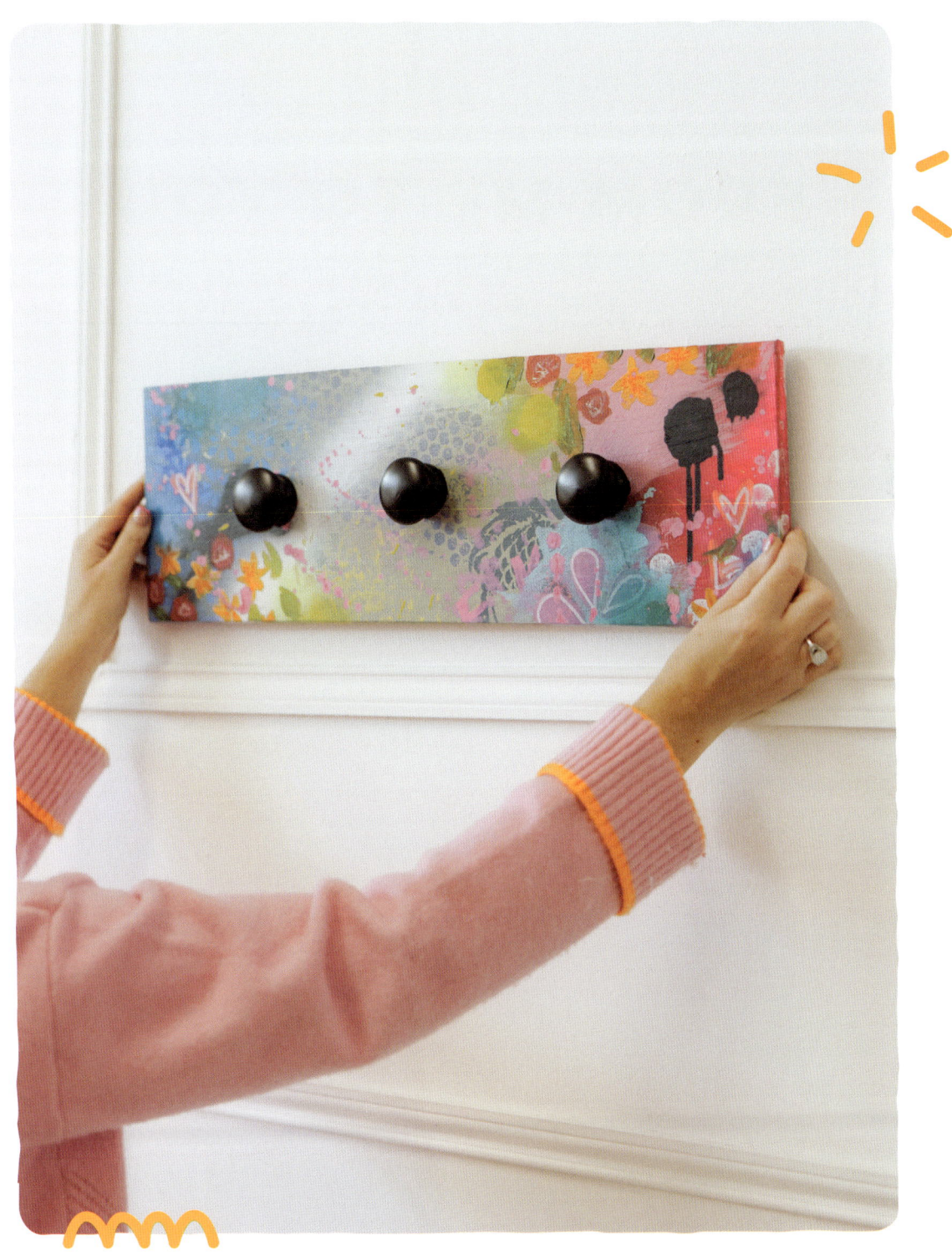

FROM ME TO YOU

So, I suppose that's it from me.

I didn't write this book in order … I rarely do anything in order. But I did save writing this part of the book until last.

I want to thank you for reading my book and hearing my story, for keeping Sean's memory alive and giving me a creative purpose

I can now say: I did it. I wrote a book!

I'm sitting here, typing away at my keyboard and feeling proud. I remember the time I lay in my bed depressed and desperate, wanting to end it all. I didn't, I got through it, I've put my passion to good use and I'm telling my tale.

I would love to wrap this book up in a nice little bow and tell you things are now exactly how I want them. I've got my happily ever after. But that's not life. I'm still on my journey and I'm still a work in progress.

I'm telling my story and making my creative mess as I go … Now, go and make yours!

I would absolutely adore it if you could share with me any of your projects inspired by this book – and maybe there's something you can relate to, or you share my views on. Please do let me know.

@gemma_longworth_diy

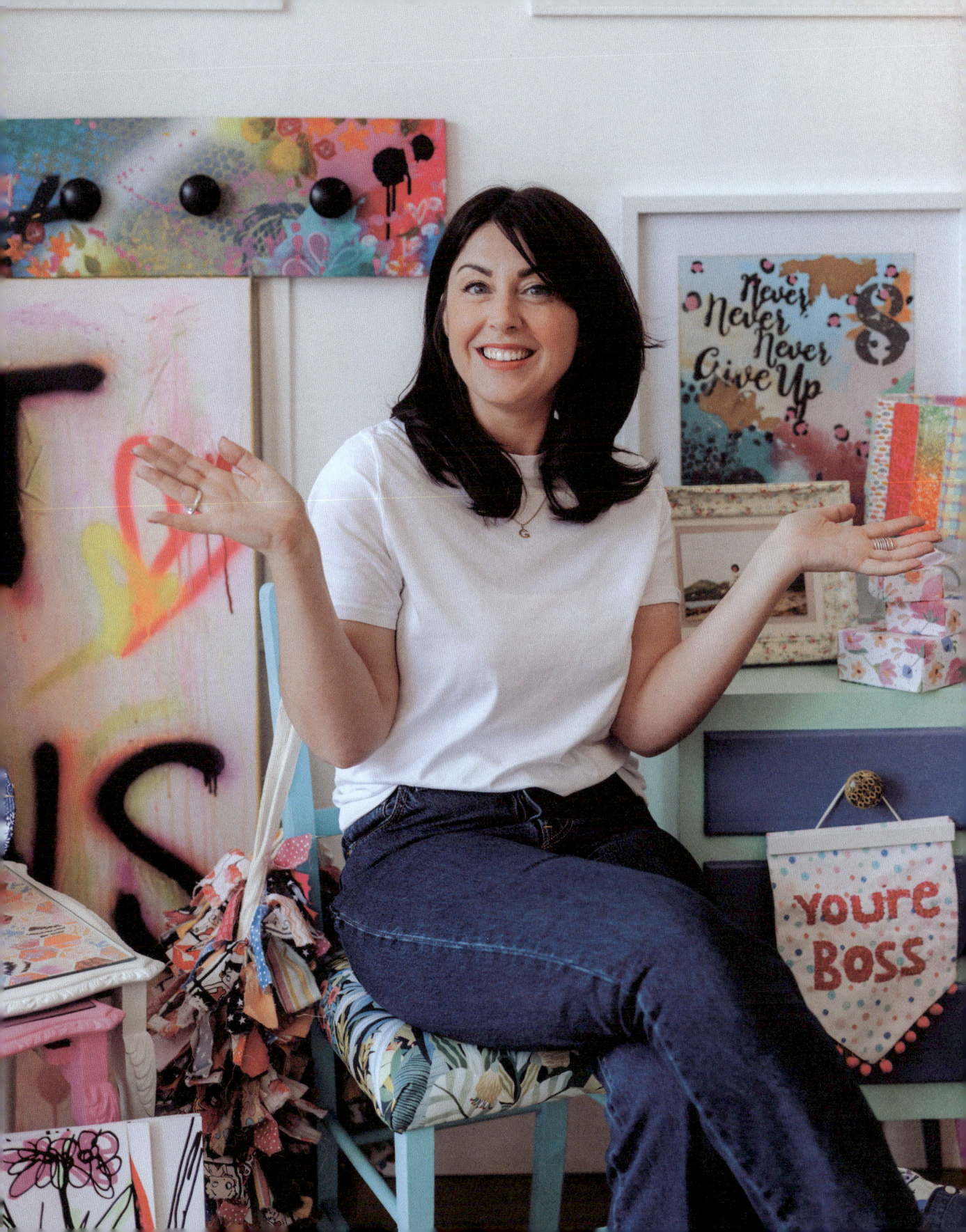

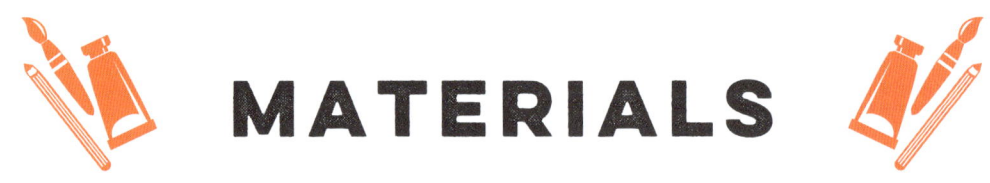

MATERIALS

Here is a list of materials that you will need to complete all of the activities within this book.

General
Sketchbook
Paper
Scissors
Glue – PVA, glue stick
Pens
Marker pens
Pencils
Eraser
Pencil sharpener
Ruler
Craft knife
Clear varnish/lacquer

Paper Crafts
Decorative paper – wrapping paper, wallpaper, tissue paper
Cardboard or corkboard
Magazines and newspapers
Blank postcards

Painting
Paints – acrylic, watercolours, oil paints, furniture paint, chalk paint
Paint brushes
Canvases
Sponge
Palette paper

Textiles
Jumbo wool
Craft wool
Ribbon
Scrap fabrics
Old clothes
Sewing-machine or hand-sewing needles
Thread
Embroidery threads
Cushion
Iron-on adhesive paper
Fabric (ideally fire retardant) for upholstery
Fabric scissors

Upcycling
Furniture – chair/small table/bedside cabinet/shelf
Picture frame
Lampshade Kit
String bag
Buttons

Waxed cord
Curtains
Stencils
Jam jar/ damaged or broken crockery
Kintsugi kit
Sandpaper (medium grit)
Sanding block
Sugar soap
Multi-surface primer
Roller and roller tray
Staple gun and staples

Clay
Air-drying clay
Shaped cookie cutters

Miscellaneous
Mirror
Bubble wrap
Spray bottle
Hair dryer

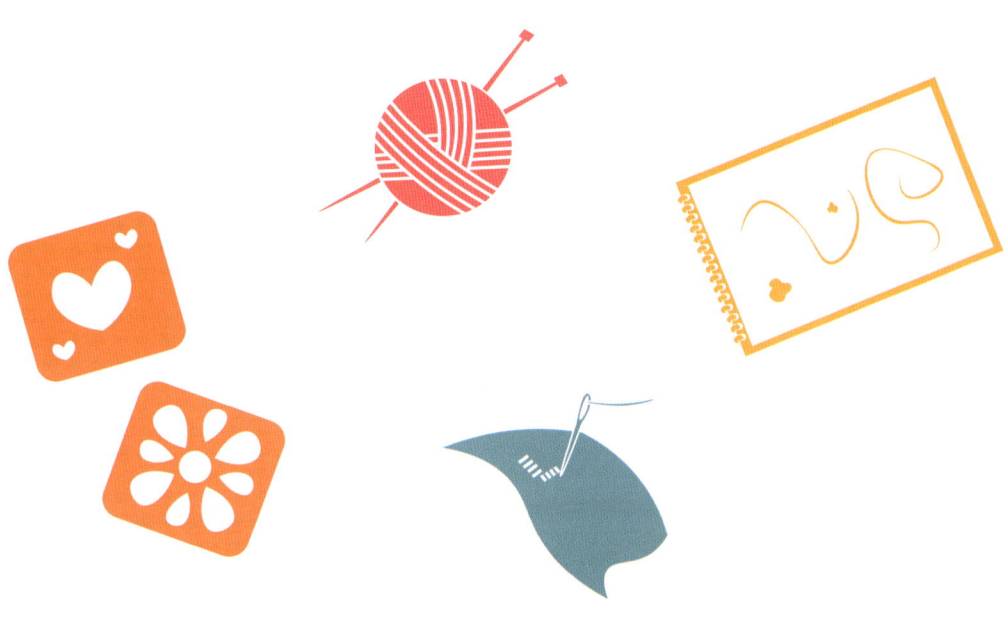

TEMPLATES

WEAR YOUR HEART ON YOUR SLEEVE

(see page 106)

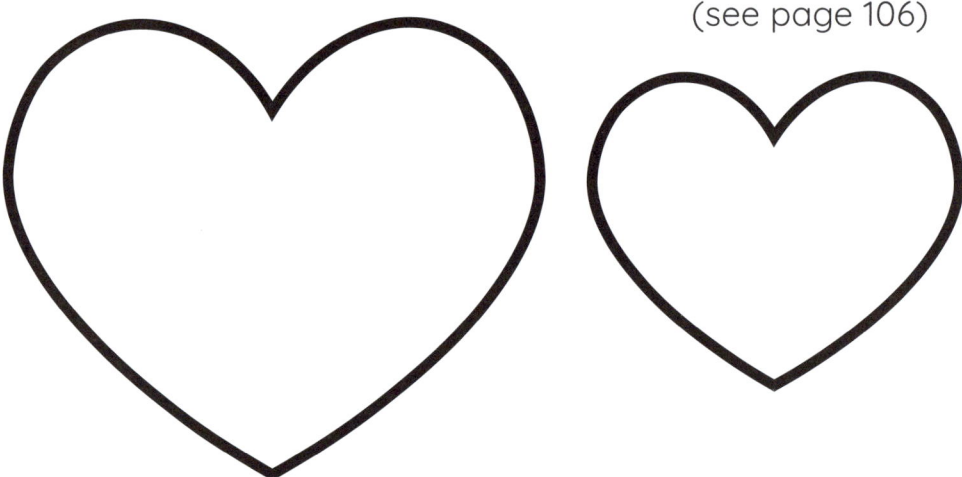

PATCHWORK DECOUPAGE TABLETOP

(see page 162)

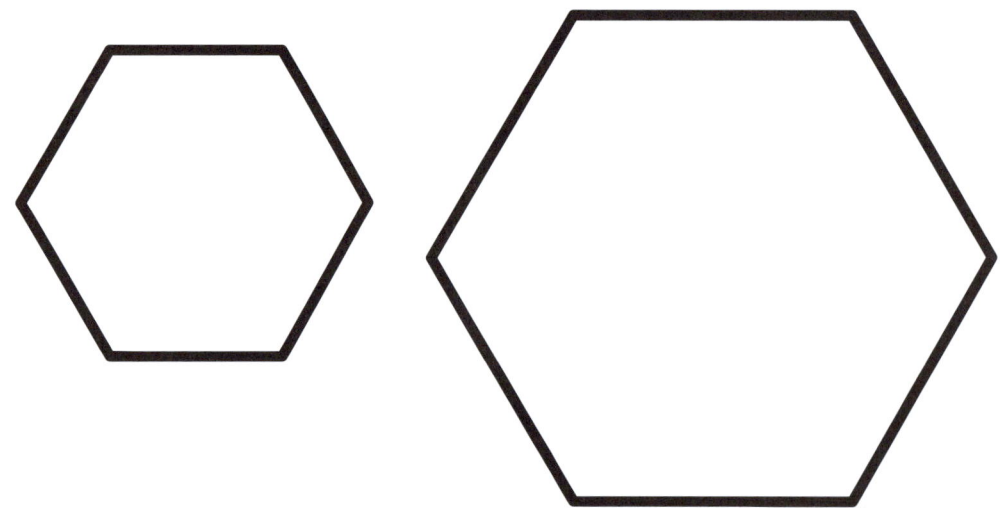

ORIGAMI GIFT BOX - BOW

(see page 54)

A

B

C

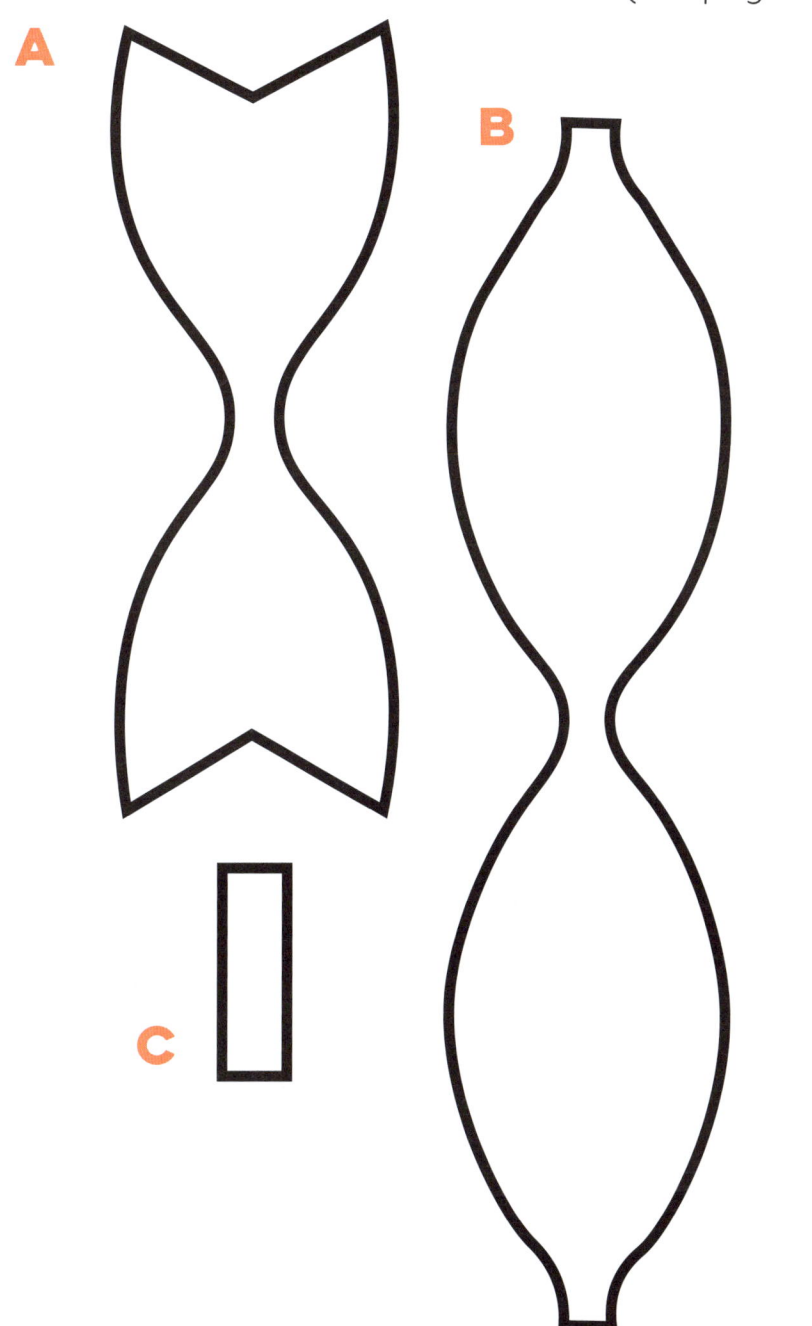

RESOURCES AND SUPPLIERS

Here is a list of resources you may find useful for further exploration into arts, crafts, upcycling and therapeutic arts. I've put together this list of websites, books, social media accounts and stores for you to gather ideas, inspiration and art materials.

Websites
Arts and crafts

★ **Pinterest** – A great platform for finding and saving ideas on DIY crafts, art projects and inspiration across multiple categories. pinterest.com

★ **Instructables** – Provides step-by-step tutorials for a wide variety of craft projects from beginner to advanced levels. instructables.com

★ **Craftsy** – Offers online classes and tutorials on various craft techniques, from knitting and quilting to painting and drawing. craftsy.com

★ **The Spruce Crafts** – Features easy-to-follow guides for home crafts, DIY and seasonal projects. thesprucecrafts.com

★ **Skillshare** – An online learning community with thousands of classes in arts, crafts and creative fields. Many courses also cover therapeutic aspects of creativity. skillshare.com

★ **Udemy** – Offers a range of affordable courses in various creative areas, including therapeutic arts, painting, crafts and DIY. udemy.com

★ **CreativeLive** – Features classes on a wide range of creative topics, including fine art, crafting and wellness-focused creative practices. creativelive.com

Therapeutic arts

★ **British Association of Art Therapists (BAAT)** – Provides extensive information about art therapy and provides resources such as publications and events relevant to the art therapy community. baat.org

★ **American Art Therapy Association (AATA)** – Offers information on art therapy and its benefits, as well as resources for professionals and individuals seeking therapy through art. arttherapy.org

★ **Mindful Art Studio** – Provides online art workshops and creative self-care resources, with a focus on mindfulness and therapeutic art practices. mindfulartstudio.com

★ **International Expressive Arts Therapy Association** – Focuses on the use of art for mental health, emotional healing and personal growth. It combines different forms of artistic expression. ieata.org

★ **Art Therapy Resources** – A collection of articles, worksheets, and resources designed for both art therapists and individuals interested in therapeutic art activities. arttherapyresources.com.au

Books

★ *The Art Therapy Sourcebook* by Cathy Malchiodi (McGraw Hill, 2006) – A comprehensive guide that explores the power of art as a therapeutic tool.

★ *Art as Therapy* by Alain de Botton and John Armstrong (Phaidon Press, 2016) – Examines how art can serve as a therapeutic medium to help people work through personal struggles.

★ *Mindful Art Therapy* by Barbara Jean Davis (Jessica Kingsley Publishers, 2015) – Combines mindfulness and art therapy practices to support emotional healing and personal wellbeing.

★ *Your Brain on Art* by Susan Magsamen and Ivy Ross (Canongate Books, 2023) – How the arts transform us.

★ *Painting Happiness* by Terry Runyan (Leaping Hare Press, 2022) – Unlock your creativity and discover the joy of watercolour painting through mindfulness.

★ *Drawing as Therapy* by The School of Life (The School of Life Press, 2021) – A collection of playful creative prompts and exercises that introduce us to the curative powers of drawing.

Art apps and tools

★ **Colour Therapy** – A social colouring app for relaxaton and mindfulness.

★ **CBT & Art Therapy** – Art therapy activities to relieve anxiety, improve self-esteem and enhance self-awareness.

★ **DIY Crafts Ideas** – A gallery app for those who want to create original things by hand.

★ **Canva** – For creating digital collages, mood boards and documents with a variety of easy-to-use templates.

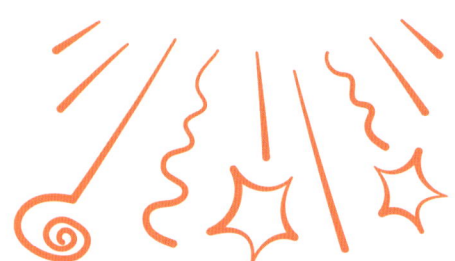

Social media accounts
Instagram & TikTok
Arts and Crafts

★ **@creativebug** – a wide range of art and craft ideas and inspiration, promoting online classes and workshops.

★ **@binebraendle** – German artist Bine Brandle showcasing endless colourful arts and craft projects

★ **@therangeartsandcrafts** – arts and crafts page for The Range store promoting customers' projects.

★ **@mrsgreenartbaby** – art teacher showcasing colourful examples of arts and craft projects for children.

★ **@the_color_file** – the colourful account of artist, author and journalist Martha Roberts.

★ **@textile_junkies** – a textile and fashion account promoting sustainability through making, creating, fixing and repairing.

★ **@gluestickgirl** – artist Lisa Truesdell showcasing her art practice using paper, glue and magic.

Upcycling

- ★ **@handsomevintage** – the colourful account of professional furniture artist Victoria Richards.

- ★ **@mucknbrass** – the fun and quirky account of Zoe Pocock, professional upcycler and charity shop campaigner.

- ★ **@sarahpetersondesign** – the vibrant account of professional upcycler, upholsterer and designer Sarah Peterson.

- ★ **@marciekdesigns** – artist, writer and designer Marcie Kobernus showcases her colourful and quirky projects.

- ★ **@nicolettetabramstencils** – a showcase of stencilling projects by designer, blogger and author Nicolette Tabram.

- ★ **@therachelhendersonstudio** – the confidently colourful account of dopamine designer Rachel Henderson.

Art

- ★ **@tiffmanuell** (art) – Australian artist Tiff Manuell showcases her painting practice and painted products.

- ★ **@sophieteaart** – Artist and influencer Sophie Tea showcases her art practice celebrating self-expression, body positivity and female empowerment.

- ★ **@lesleygrainger** – the inspirational account of colourful abstract artist Lesley Grainger.

- ★ **@aceagrams** – the official social media account for the Arts Council England.

- ★ **@thelittleartistsroom** – art education projects for children, supporting teachers and parents with ideas and inspiration.

- ★ **@lizmurphystudio** – a photo gallery for abstract artist, designer and art coach Liz Murphy.

- ★ **@katiestraus_art** – a photo gallery showcasing the work of abstract floral artist Katie Straus.

- ★ **@brittleeart** – colourful abstract, expressive paintings by artist Brittany Lee Howard.

- ★ **@tipperleyhill** – artist duo Roz Berkeley-Hill and Abi Tippetts showcase their works of art, window painting and workshops.

★ **@jessicaslackstudio** – colourful abstract artworks inspired by nature by artist Jessica Slack.

★ **@artisticsideoflife_** – the account of collage artist Maya Land showcasing her quirky and playful collage art.

★ **@windsorandnewton** – promote a wide range of artist's materials, tutorials and inspiring artworks.

★ **@dalerrowney1783** – featuring professional art supplies, creative techniques, ideas and inspiration.

★ **@baat_org** – highlights the work of the British Association of Art Therapists.

★ **@doodlegems** – graphic design and illustration prompting joy and positivity through colourful illustrations.

Suppliers
UK Arts and Crafts Material Suppliers

★ **Hobbycraft** – hobbycraft.co.uk
One of the largest arts and crafts retailers in the UK, offering a wide range of materials, from painting supplies to fabric and knitting materials, both online and in stores.

★ **Cass Art** – cassart.co.uk
With multiple stores across the UK, Cass Art specializes in fine art supplies, offering everything from canvas and paint to sketching tools. There is also an online store.

★ **Fred Aldous** – fredaldous.co.uk
Based in Manchester, Fred Aldous offers a wide variety of art and craft supplies, including materials for drawing, painting, printmaking and DIY crafts. They ship across the UK.

★ **The Range** – therange.co.uk
This retailer stocks a large selection of arts and crafts materials, from canvases and paints to knitting and sewing supplies, with many physical stores and online shopping.

★ **Art Discount** – artdiscount.co.uk
A UK-based online store offering discounted prices on a range of art supplies, including paints, drawing tools and craft kits for all ages.

★ **B&Q** – diy.com
A British multinational DIY and home improvement retail company, offering a wide range of products for home renovation, gardening and interior design.

USA arts and crafts material suppliers

★ **Michaels** – michaels.com
One of the largest craft stores in the USA, Michaels carries a wide selection of art supplies, craft materials, framing services and project kits for every skill level.

★ **Joann Fabrics & Crafts** – joann.com
Joann specializes in fabrics and sewing supplies but also carries a wide range of art and crafting materials, including yarn, paper crafts, and tools for DIY projects.

★ **Blick Art Materials** – dickblick.com
Blick is one of the most trusted suppliers for professional artists and students, offering a comprehensive selection of art materials for painting, drawing, sculpture and more.

★ **Jerry's Artarama** – jerrysartarama.com
A large supplier of fine art materials, Jerry's Artarama offers high-quality products for painting, drawing, printmaking and other crafts, with online shopping and nationwide shipping.

★ **Paper Source** – papersource.com
Specializes in paper crafts, offering unique stationery, paper and crafting tools for creative projects like scrapbooking, card making and journalling.

★ **Hobby Lobby** – hobbylobby.com
A large US-based craft store chain offering supplies for a wide range of arts and crafts, including painting, floral arrangements, needlework and DIY home projects.

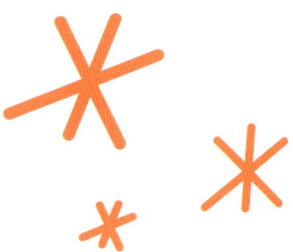

ACKNOWLEDGEMENTS

This process of writing this book has been quite the journey for me. As someone who has dyslexia I never thought it would be possible to write a book. It's certainly been a challenge, often a struggle and some days a burden. But I'm so pleased I stuck with it.

I wanted to do this for myself to prove that I can do anything if I put my mind to it.

This book wouldn't have happened without the support of people I'm lucky to have around me.

My Mum, who is there for me no matter what, for bringing me lunch when I wasn't able to leave the house because I was so bogged down with work.

For my boyfriend and my friends who have listened to me talk about this book for the last year. I'm sure they will be as relieved as I am that it's finally written and we can all talk about something else.

For DML Talent and Watkins publishing for believing that I could do this and encouraging me every step of the way.

For all the Hidden Gems who are living with the loss of their loved ones. I hope the activities within this book made your days a little brighter and lighter.

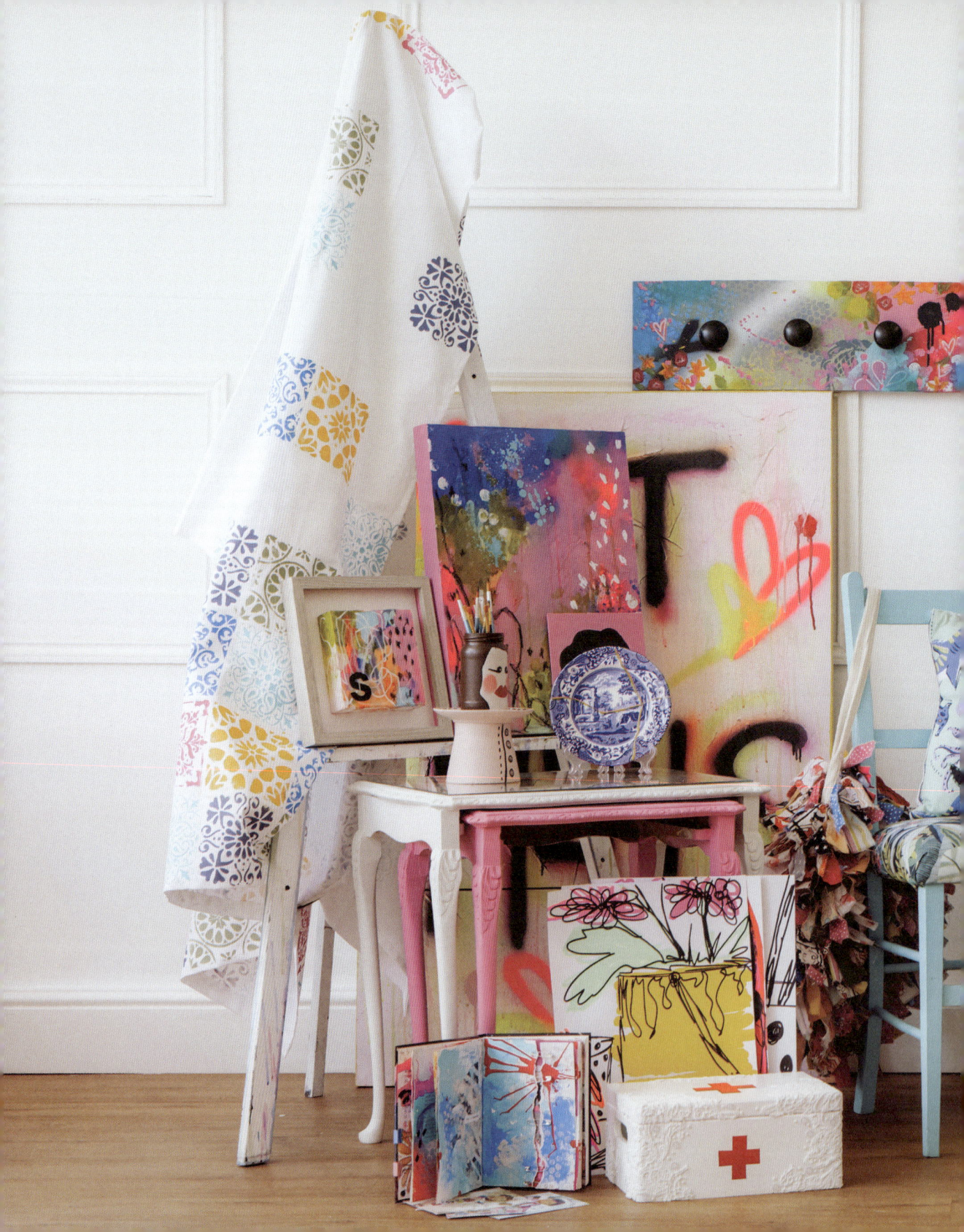

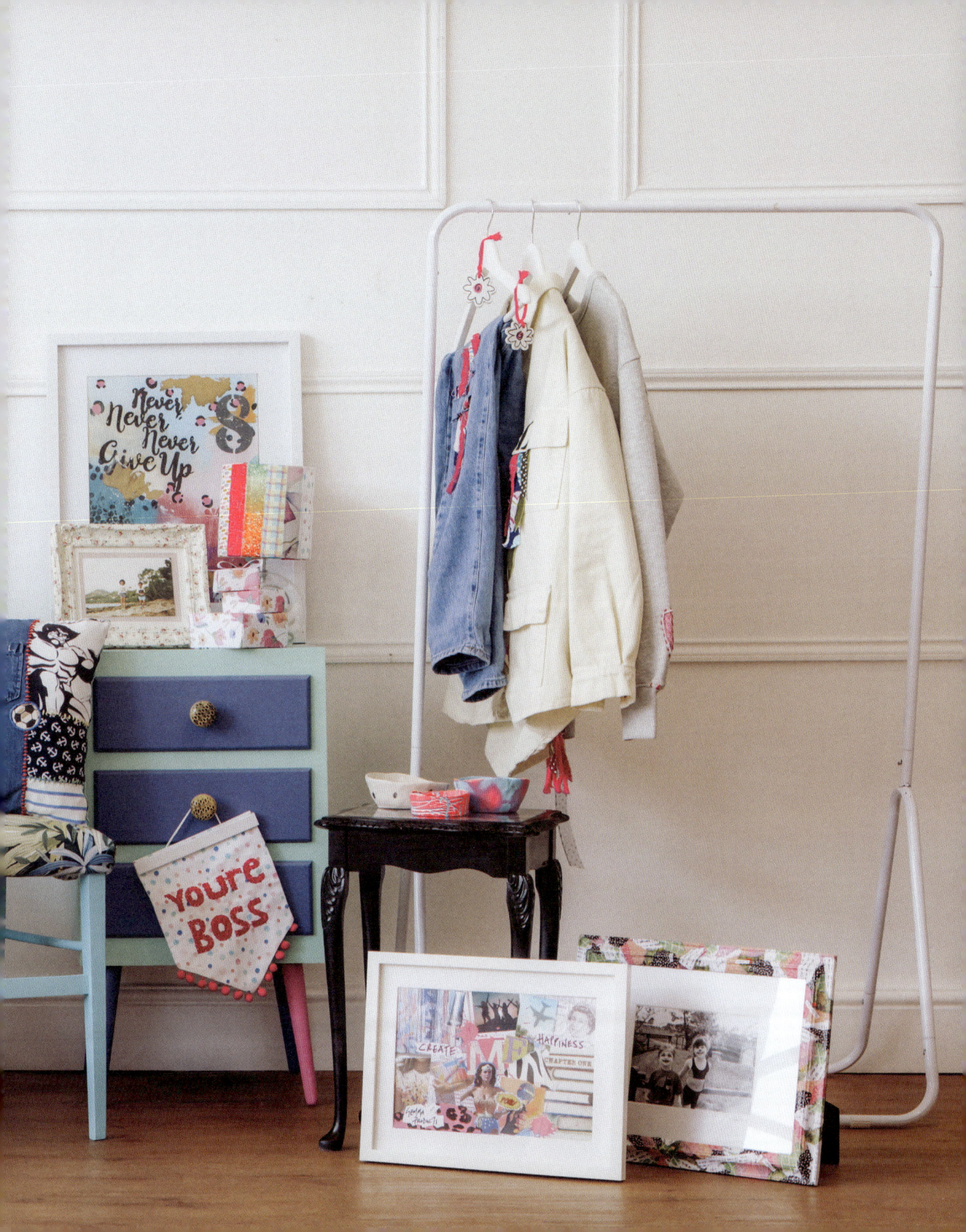